The Quality and Outcomes Framework

QOF – TRANSFORMING GENERAL PRACTICE

Edited by

STEPHEN GILLAM

General Practitioner
Director, Undergraduate Public Health Teaching
University of Cambridge

and

A NIROSHAN SIRIWARDENA

Professor of Primary and Prehospital Health Care, University of Lincoln
General Practitioner
Editor, Quality in Primary Care

Foreword by

Iona Heath

President
Royal College of General Practitioners

Radcliffe Publishing
Oxford • New York

Radcliffe Publishing Ltd
18 Marcham Road
Abingdon
Oxon OX14 1AA
United Kingdom

www.radcliffepublishing.com

Electronic catalogue and worldwide online ordering facility.

British Library Cataloguing in Publication Data

A catalogue record for this book is available from the British Library.

ISBN-13: 978 184619 456 6

The paper used for the text pages of this book is FSC certified. FSC (The Forest Stewardship Council) is an international network to promote responsible management of the world's forests.

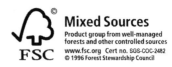

Mixed Sources
Product group from well-managed forests and other controlled sources
www.fsc.org Cert no. SGS-COC-2482
© 1996 Forest Stewardship Council

Typeset by KnowledgeWorks Global Ltd, Chennai, India
Printed and bound by TJI Digital, Padstow, Cornwall, UK

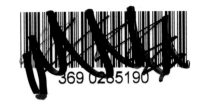

The Quality and Outcomes Framework

Contents

Foreword

The Quality and Outcomes Framework (QOF) has deeply divided UK general practitioners (GPs). Some feel that, at last, general practitioners who provide a high standard of care are being proportionately rewarded; others appreciate the grounding of the QOF within the realm of evidence-based medicine and the step change in practice computer systems that it has triggered.

Most profit-sharing partners are happy with the increased income that it brought, but those in fixed salary positions, along with other members of the practice team, may justifiably resent the unequal distribution of the extra income.

However, many other general practitioners have found themselves feeling compromised by a system that they find reductive and that makes no allowance for the profound differences between individual patients, even when they are assigned the same diagnostic label. Primary care makes its contribution to the health of population by integrating care around the needs of particular individuals not by focusing on single diseases.

Biomedical evidence is in a constant state of flux, with successive trials moderating the findings of earlier ones, and yet the QOF risks ossifying the evidence base for at least a year. Some argue that it may have the effect of reducing the responsibility of doctors to think, to question and to judge wisely. The contributors to this important book examine in detail the published evidence on the impact of the QOF so far.

In his 2010 Bradford Hill Lecture at the London School of Hygiene and Tropical Medicine, Professor Sander Greenland raised fundamental concerns that contemporary medical research is based on hopelessly over-simplified biological and mathematical models. He asked profound questions about the state of the 'evidence' on which the QOF is based which should give even its most enthusiastic supporters at least some small whisper of concern.

In her book *Science and Poetry*, the philosopher Mary Midgley writes:

> Out of this fascination with new power there arises our current huge
> expansion of technology, much of it useful, much not, and the sheer

size of it (as we now see) dangerously wasteful of resources. It is hard for us to break out of this circle of increasing needs because our age is remarkably preoccupied with the vision of continually improving means rather than saving ourselves trouble by reflecting on ends.

The QOF provides a perfect illustration of this point. We have become obsessed with the means and have neglected to consider our ends. How should we live? When should we die? How does the normative aspiration for a long and healthy life rank alongside the multitude of other human hopes and aspirations? How can we best care for those facing the intrusions and distresses of chronic disease?

I commend this book and applaud its determination to scrutinise every aspect of the Quality and Outcomes Framework – good and bad and in between.

Iona Heath
President, RCGP
August 2010

About the editors

Stephen Gillam is a GP in Luton and Director of Undergraduate Public Health Teaching at the University of Cambridge. Previously, he was director of primary care at the King's Fund where he was heavily involved in charting the impact of health policy under New Labour. He is an honorary consultant at the Cambridgeshire Primary Care Trust and a visiting professor at the University of Bedfordshire.

A Niroshan Siriwardena is professor of primary and pre hospital healthcare at the University of Lincoln. He is a GP with research interests centred on quality improvement in primary and pre hospital care. He is editor of *Quality in Primary Care* and an executive member of the *European Forum for Primary Care*.

List of contributors

CHAPTER 2

Martin Roland is a professor of health services research at Cambridge University. Previously, he was a professor of general practice at Manchester University for 17 years. He has been a practicing GP for over 30 years, and in 2002/03 was one of the academic advisers to the government and BMA negotiating teams on the QOF.

CHAPTER 3

Stephen Campbell is a health services researcher and senior research fellow at the University of Manchester. His research interests focus on quality of care in general practice, and he currently co-leads the external contractor group (with Helen Lester) advising NICE on developing the QOF.

Helen Lester is a GP and professor of primary care at the University of Manchester. She has been working as an academic adviser on the QOF since 2005 and currently co-leads the external contractor group (with Stephen Campbell) advising NICE on developing the QOF.

CHAPTER 4

Nicholas Steel is interested in health services research and improving the quality of healthcare. After graduating from medical school in 1988, he worked as a GP in the United Kingdom, Australia and New Zealand. He trained in public health and health policy in Norfolk, Cambridge and RAND Health in California.

Sara Willems is a post-doctoral fellow at the department of general practice and primary healthcare at Ghent University. Her research focuses on the social gradient in medical healthcare use, the accessibility of the Belgian healthcare system and the role of primary healthcare in tackling health inequalities.

CHAPTER 5

Anna Dixon is a director of policy at the King's Fund. She has researched and published widely on healthcare funding and policy. She was previously a lecturer at the London School of Economics and worked in the Strategy Unit at the Department of Health.

Artak Khachatryan is a researcher in health policy at the King's Fund. He graduated from Yerevan State Medical University (Armenia) with a PhD in surgery. He was awarded a PhD in public health and epidemiology at University College London where he worked as a researcher. He also worked as a clinical research fellow at London School of Hygiene and Tropical Medicine.

Tammy Boyce is a research fellow in public health at the King's Fund. She was a senior research fellow at the Strategic Review of Health Inequalities in England. She is an author of *Health, Risk and News: The MMR Vaccine and the Media* (Peter Lang; 2007) and an editor of *Climate Change and the Media: Global Crises and the Media* (Peter Lang Pub Inc; 2009).

CHAPTER 6

Maria Kordowicz holds degrees in psychology, mental health studies and public policy and management and presently works as a senior healthcare manager in East London. Maria's PhD is an exploration of the organisational meanings of quality and performance in general practice, supervised by Dr Mark Ashworth.

Mark Ashworth graduated in medicine from Southampton University and after a short dalliance with tropical medicine has been working as a GP in an inner city practice in South London since 1987. He gained his doctorate in 2004 and was subsequently appointed clinical senior lecturer at King's College London.

CHAPTER 7

Kath Checkland qualified as a GP in 1991 and worked as a GP partner for 12 years. In 1999, she returned to academic work, obtaining an MA in 2001 and a PhD in 2005. She now works 2 days a week as a salaried GP and 3 days a week as a clinical senior lecturer. Her research focuses upon the impact of health policy on primary care organisations.

Stephen Harrison is a professor of social policy at the University of Manchester, where he heads the organisational research programme within the National Primary Care Research & Development Centre. His most recent book is *The Politics of Healthcare in Britain* with Ruth McDonald (Sage; 2008).

CHAPTER 8

Chantal Simon has been a GP since 2005 and is currently a part-time GP Partner in Bournemouth with day-to-day experience of working with the QOF. She is a co-author of the *Handbook of Practice Management* and has written on the QOF and GP Contract in that capacity.

Anna Morton is an experienced practice manager. She has been practice manager at Whiteparish Surgery but now works as practice manager at Avon Valley Practice, both in Wiltshire. Her day-to-day work involves organisation and delivery of the QOF.

CHAPTER 9

Patricia Wilkie is a social scientist with a particular interest in the patient perspective. This is reflected in her academic work and in voluntary work with the medical Royal Colleges, the Academy of Medical Royal Colleges, disease organisations, charities and government committees. She is currently president of National Association for Patient Participation (NAPP).

CHAPTER 10

Stephen Peckham is a reader in health policy in the Department of Health Services Research and Policy, London School of Hygiene and Tropical Medicine. His main research interests are in health policy analysis, inter-agency collaboration, primary care, public health and public involvement. Apart from his work examining the QOF, he is also currently exploring the role of general practice in public health, patient choice policy in the United Kingdom and how people with long-term conditions are engaged in commissioning health services.

Andrew Wallace is a research fellow in the Department of Health Services Research and Policy, London School of Hygiene and Tropical Medicine. He works on research projects that explore innovations in the design and delivery of primary care, including the development of polysystems and the growing use of financial incentives and how these impact on quality of care and health inequalities.

CHAPTER 11

Barbara Starfield is University Distinguished Professor of Health Policy at the Johns Hopkins University. Understanding the effectiveness and equity of health services, especially primary care and specialty care, are her foci. Other areas of interest are measures of morbidity, including casemix, as they relate to the need for, use of and quality of services.

Dee Mangin is a New Zealand family physician who is currently an associate professor and director of the Primary Care Research Group at the Christchurch School of Medicine, University of Otago. Her interests are rational prescribing and the influence of science, policy and commerce on the nature of care.

List of figures

List of tables

List of boxes

PART I

Background to the Quality and Outcomes Framework

CHAPTER 1

Introduction: development, impact and implications

Steve Gillam and A Niroshan Siriwardena

SUMMARY

The Quality and Outcomes Framework (QOF), introduced into UK general practice in 2004, is unarguably the most comprehensive national primary care pay-for-performance (P4P) scheme in the world. A natural experiment on such a large scale provides extraordinary possibilities for research, analysis and reflection. This book is an attempt to make use of this unique opportunity to explore the scheme in depth.

In this introductory chapter, we describe the contents of each section and how they fit together. Although each chapter stands alone, together they construct a more coherent picture of the QOF. The book considers the origins of the QOF and how it is being developed further; it seeks to summarise and analyse the research undertaken on its impact, including potential unintended or adverse consequences and the gaps in evidence. It provides a viewpoint from practitioners and patients implementing and experiencing the scheme. Finally, it reflects on the lessons for P4P and primary care in the United Kingdom in future and in other settings. In doing so, contributors scrutinise the evidence from the varying perspectives of academic, practitioner, service user and policy analyst.

We hope this book provides practitioners, politicians and policy makers with emerging evidence and critical reflection to inform the development of primary care and P4P systems in the United Kingdom and beyond.

Key points
- Politicians and commissioners of services are seeking mechanisms that will consistently deliver high-quality care.

- The QOF, the most comprehensive national primary care P4P scheme in the world, provides a unique opportunity for research, analysis and reflection.
- This chapter provides an overview of the different sections and chapters of the book and how they construct a coherent picture of the QOF.
- Practitioners, politicians and policy makers should use the emerging evidence and critical reflection on this to inform the development of primary care and P4P systems.

INTRODUCTION

Health services are under ever greater pressure to provide high-quality care that is safe, effective, efficient and timely and where patients' needs and experiences are heeded.[1,2] The pace of organisational change within the UK National Health Service (NHS) over the last two decades to try and meet these needs has been bewildering. Yet for all that, the rituals and routines of day-to-day general practice have seemed, at least on the surface, to endure without significant alteration. By contrast, the impact of the QOF has, arguably, exceeded that of any other policy development since the Family Doctors' Charter of 1966. This huge national experiment in performance-related pay has understandably attracted much international attention and is likely to continue to do so.[3,4]

The Griffiths reforms of the mid-1980s first introduced private-sector management methods into the NHS.[5] These methods borrowed on systems theory developed at the Rand corporation that espoused markets, performance indicators, benchmarking, targets and incentives. Alan Enthoven advocated applying these ideas to healthcare; they were reflected in reforms introduced by the conservative government under Margaret Thatcher and the labour administration of Tony Blair that followed.[6] The QOF has developed within the context of the NHS' quasi-market that seeks to separate purchasers ('commissioners') and providers of care. In historical terms, the QOF represents a high water mark in the onward march of what Harrison has elsewhere termed 'scientific managerialism' in healthcare.[7] The QOF also provides commissioners with albeit crude tools for comparing providers as they seek to break the monopolistic stranglehold of traditional general practice in the UK primary healthcare sector.

Since its introduction in 2004, the effects of the QOF on quality of care have been the subject of pained debate. Six years on, that debate is being informed by an accumulating body of research. As the political and economic environment in the United Kingdom herald further organisational disruption, searching analysis of this evidence is timely. Through an international cast of expert contributors, this book seeks to provide just such a multifaceted review.

STRUCTURE

Part I focuses on the background to the QOF, how it was initially conceived and how it continues to be maintained and developed. Martin Roland describes how the QOF emerged from previous policy initiatives that promoted improvement through clinical audit, within a system of quality and accountability known as clinical governance. He describes how P4P dramatically improved attainments when it was introduced for cervical screening and childhood immunisation, and the influence of a forerunner of the QOF. He provides a fascinating insider's account of the context for introduction of the framework as well as describing the negotiations and those involved.

Helen Lester and Stephen Campbell further examine the origins of the QOF framework dating back to antecedents that attempted to promote evidence-based primary care. Much development of performance indicators was undertaken in the National Primary Care Research and Development Centre, and they describe how that work progressed. The metamorphosis of what began as a scheme for quality and improvement into a regulated, contractual framework now requires burgeoning technical support for development and implementation of 'feasible, valid, reliable and piloted "QOFable" clinical indicators'.

Part II summarises, reviews and analyses the research findings: positive, negative and consequences yet unknown or uncertain.

Partly because of its scale and complexity, the impact of the QOF will always be hard to quantify. Nick Steel and Sara Willems, in their broad ranging review of research on the QOF help to identify the impact of the QOF and its effects over and above the preceding secular trends. They explore issues of equity and cost effectiveness arising from the QOF. They also analyse the nature of the evidence, the strengths and flaws inherent in the research and gaps that remain.

A central rationale for the QOF was the need to reduce longstanding variations in the quality of primary care provision. In particular, successive reports had highlighted poor-quality care in more deprived, urban areas.[8,9] Maria Kordowicz and Mark Ashworth explore the notion that the QOF may have increased the quality of chronic disease management or narrowed inequalities in health and healthcare delivery or whether this is an artefact of the system. They discuss whether improvements are more apparent than real – the product of better and more comprehensive data collection. They also discuss the issue of 'gaming' and data manipulation.

Focusing their attention on population-wide health improvement and reduction of inequalities, Anna Dixon and Artak Khachatryan examine differences in performance between practices in areas with the worst health and deprivation indicators and those in other areas. They go on to discuss the strength of evidence of narrowing in the equity gap and whether this can be attributed with certainty to the QOF. They argue that the QOF should explicitly address health inequalities in the future development of QOF indicators.

In essence, judgements on the QOF involve balancing sensitive evaluation of the health gains against assessment of its costs, many of which are hard to quantify. Just how hard is apparent from the contribution by Kath Checkland and Steve Harrison. In their analysis of the effects of the QOF on the front line of practice and organisation, they find that greater specialisation among practice nurses has, in turn, promoted extension of the role of other cadres such as healthcare assistants in some practices. They explore how new roles and hierarchies have been created and accepted within practices and how this is affecting morale and motivation.

Part III focuses on practical aspects of the QOF. Chantal Simon and Anna Morton demonstrate how practices can approach the QOF and succeed in achieving high scores through forward planning and good organisation. They also discuss how practices need to make decisions about which targets to pursue as these become progressively harder to achieve and give examples of how practice teams should approach the QOF in a pragmatic way.

Surprisingly, little is known of what service users, the most important stake-holders, think, and several authors comment that there has been little substantive research on the impact of the QOF from the users' perspective. This point is developed by Patricia Wilkie. In her chapter, she discusses what patients want from their care and focuses on the importance of the relationship between patient and practitioner. She restates the importance of a 'whole person' approach and the fragmenting effect of the QOF on continuity and trust. She explores what patients understand by the QOF and the importance of explaining why QOF data are being collected to patients. The QOF has begun another revolution in the assessment of primary healthcare quality through the incorporation of systematic patient feedback. Despite this, many patients probably do not understand the financial framework that general practice operates within and the effect of payments on the actions of the professionals that care for them.

Part IV reflects on P4P within and outside the QOF: its successes, failures and lessons for others. Stephen Peckham and Andrew Wallace show us the broad canvas of international evidence on P4P schemes. It is striking how much the empirical research they amass already relates to the QOF. They argue that although P4P schemes can affect clinical behaviour and processes, its impact on quality more broadly defined (such as patient experience or outcomes) is less clear. Their analysis shows how many of the concerns arising from implementation of this new scheme were predictable on the basis of previous research on P4P.

Finally, Barbara Starfield and Dee Mangin provide an international perspective on P4P and reflect on whether the QOF supports or detracts from those features of primary care systems that underlie their success in promoting health. They question the nature of the QOF's evidence base and whether such schemes can address co-morbidities and the individual variation in patients presenting to general practice.

CONCLUSIONS

Many features of the system within which the QOF operates, such as the internal market, competition and regulation, challenge the philosophies of improvement pioneers of the past. Deming's five 'deadly diseases' – lack of constancy of purpose, emphasising profits and targets, changing management, relying on annual ratings of performance and using visible figures only – are rife in the NHS today.[10] We revisit these ideas in the last chapter to discuss whether the current framework is geared to improve quality of primary care and patient outcomes.

For all those interested in the development of primary care, in the United Kingdom and internationally, these contributions will provide much to reflect upon. The QOF is a natural experiment in progress; verdicts even at this stage of its evolution must be qualified. The QOF is being used in other countries to compare systems' performance,[11] even attempting to improve on the indicators used[12]; some are considering the potential for its adoption.[13] A change of government presages further changes to general practitioners' contracts. Politicians and policy makers should be minded to heed the emerging evidence.[14]

REFERENCES

1. Institute of Medicine. *Crossing the Quality Chasm: a new health system for the 21st century*. Washington, DC: National Academy Press; 2001.
2. Darzi of Denham AD. *High Quality Care for All: NHS next stage review final report*. London: Stationery Office; 2008.
3. Roland M. Pay-for-Performance: too much of a good thing? A conversation with Martin Roland. Interview by Robert Galvin. *Health Aff (Millwood)*. 2006; **25**: w412–w419.
4. Shekelle P. New contract for general practitioners. *BMJ*. 2003; **326**: 457–8.
5. Griffiths R. *NHS Management Inquiry Report*. London: NHS Management Inquiry; 1983.
6. Curtis A. *The Trap – what happened to our dream of freedom?* London: BBC; 2007.
7. Harrison S, Moran M, Wood B. Policy emergence and policy convergence: the case of 'Scientific Bureaucratic Medicine'. *Br J Polit Int Relations*. 2002; **4**: 1–24.
8. Department of Health and Social Security. *Inequalities in Health: report of a research working group*. London: Department of Health and Social Security;1980.
9. Acheson D. *Independent Inquiry into Inequalities in Health Report*. London: Stationery Office;1998.
10. Deming WS. *Out of the Crisis*. Cambridge, MA: MIT; 1962.
11. Crosson JC, Ohman-Strickland PA, Campbell S, *et al*. A comparison of chronic illness care quality in US and UK family medicine practices prior to pay-for-performance initiatives. *Fam Pract*. 2009; **26**: 510–16.
12. Mabotuwana T, Warren J, Elley R, *et al*. Use of interval based quality indicators in blood pressure management to enhance quality of pay-for-performance incentives – comparison to two indicators from the Quality and Outcomes Framework. *Qual Prim Care*. 2010; **18**: 93–101.
13. van den Heuvel HG, Mand P, Heim S, *et al*. Views of German general practitioners on the clinical indicators of the British Quality and Outcomes Framework: a qualitative study. *Qual Prim Care*. 2010; **18**: 85–92.
14. Department of Health. *Equity and Excellence: liberating the NHS*. London: Department of Health; 2010.

CHAPTER 2

Where did the Quality and Outcomes Framework come from?

Martin Roland

SUMMARY

This chapter describes the origins of the Quality and Outcomes Framework (QOF) and discusses how the initial attempts to incentivise quality developed from medical audit, clinical governance and target payments for childhood immunisations and cervical cytology. It goes on to describe how the pay-for-performance scheme was negotiated, how the quality indicators were first developed and how the payment structure was agreed upon.

Key points

- The QOF developed from early attempts at introducing quality improvement through medical audit and clinical governance.
- Incentives were successfully introduced in 1990 in the form of target payments for childhood immunisations and cervical screening.
- Indicators were developed from national guidance or clear professional consensus, and many had been tested in an early local P4P scheme.
- Payments were based on estimated workload for the care involved.

ORIGINS

In 1986, the UK Department of Health tried to introduce a 'Good Practice Allowance' into general practice, which would have offered financial incentives for practices that provided high-quality care. This was dismissed by the British Medical Association (BMA) as 'political and provocative, prepared by a policy unit whose main contact seemed to have been with philosophers, privateers and trendy professors'.[1] Yet, by 2001, the BMA's negotiators were enthusiastic about negotiating a remuneration package that was dependent on measuring quality of care across a wide range of conditions. This was a major change from 15 years before. Those intervening years had seen a substantial cultural change that led general practitioners (GPs) to accept that a substantial amount of their pay would be related to quality of care.

The first significant change in the attitudes and practice of GPs resulted from the introduction of audit as a requirement of the 1990 GP Contract. Initially, audits were patchy and rarely carried out across whole geographical areas; it was also uncommon for the audit cycle to be completed. Locally, audit was championed by small numbers of enthusiasts who often became chairs of local medical audit advisory groups. These groups began to develop more systematic approaches to audit in general practice,[2] and during that decade, audit was also included as a requirement for vocational training in general practice. By the end of the decade, clinical audit was becoming a regular activity in many practices.[3] The gradual development of audit during the 1990s familiarised GPs with the idea of looking more carefully at the care they were providing. Research studies showed widespread deficiencies in quality of care[4]; when GPs measured care in their own practices, they found that care could be improved.

A further change introduced into the 1990 GP Contract was the first UK experiment in pay-for-performance (P4P): the introduction of financial incentives to achieve targets for childhood immunisation and cervical cytology. These incentives were associated with a substantial rise in achievement in these clinical areas, especially among previously low performing practices. This led to a progressive reduction of inequality in the delivery of care, with practices in socio-economically deprived areas steadily improving their performance in comparison with practices in affluent areas.[5,6] The introduction of these incentives in 1990 also led many general practices to invest in their first computers, since it was difficult to achieve the targets without an effective recall system. Over the next decade, computers were increasingly used for prescribing and then for clinical records. Financial support for practice information technology (IT) systems from the National Health Service (NHS) started to provide the electronic infrastructure upon which the QOF would subsequently be based.

The 1990s saw two more significant changes. First, the health promotion banding scheme was introduced, which rewarded GPs for the first time for systematic data collection in relation to preventive strategies around smoking and conditions such as hypertension. Second, in 1996, a sustained quality allowance (SQA) was introduced, which rewarded practices for using a formulary and for systematically managing some chronic diseases. Also, practices would not achieve the SQA unless they also achieved their immunisation targets. Interestingly, training practices were automatically awarded the allowance, on the grounds that they already had a form of quality accreditation.

In the late 1990s, the New Labour government launched a plethora of initiatives to improve quality of care across the NHS.[7] Some of these fell under the umbrella of 'clinical governance', which emphasised a more systematic local approach to audit. They ran in parallel with a developing national infrastructure being developed to support quality improvement: National Service Frameworks, the National Institute for Health and Clinical Excellence (NICE) and new appraisal systems for NHS doctors (*see* Figure 2.1).

By the end of the decade, doctors had become accustomed to measuring the quality of their care and working out ways of improving it. They were also accustomed to using computers in their practices. Then, in 2000, the prime minister announced that there was to be an increase in NHS funding to bring the United Kingdom to mid-European levels in terms of expenditure as a proportion of gross domestic product (GDP). This was because of increasing public concern about the quality of healthcare in the United Kingdom. Specialists saw this as a bonanza. The acute sector never had difficulty spending money, and the challenge for GPs and their negotiators was to ensure that some of this new money would flow into primary care, the locus of increasing provision. It was clear that GPs would have to deliver something substantial in return for additional investment, even though

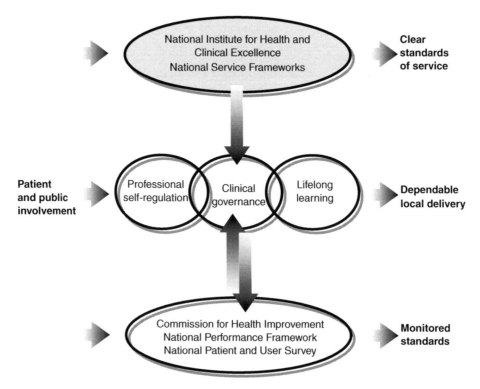

FIGURE 2.1 Quality-Improvement Framework[8] [Commission for Health Improvement (CHI) is now the Care Quality Commission]

there was general agreement that recruitment problems and poor morale in general practice would require an overall pay increase for GPs. GP negotiators decided that what they could deliver in return for increased investment in primary care was improved quality. So, they went as willing partners into the negotiations that produced the QOF.

NEGOTIATING THE QOF

Negotiations took place as a new GP Contract was drawn up in 2002 and 2003. They were negotiations between the employer (in this case the NHS Confederation representing the Department of Health) and the trades union (the BMA representing GPs). Dr John Chisholm led for the BMA as chair of the GP Committee (GPC), and Dr Tony Snell led the employer side. Dr Snell was an ex-GP and a medical adviser in East Kent. Observers were present from the health departments of the four devolved nations, England, Scotland, Wales and Northern Ireland. There were normally about 15 people present at these negotiating sessions. The majority of those present were GPs, on both sides of the negotiating table.

A group of expert advisers were invited to take part by both teams. They attended negotiating meetings over a period of around 12 months but did much of the work outside the meetings. Dr Colin Hunter [ex-chair Scottish Royal College of General Practitioners (RCGPs) Council] and Martin Roland (professor of general practice, University of Manchester) led the advisers and were present at most negotiating sessions. They were joined by Dr Malcolm Campbell (senior lecturer in general practice, University of Glasgow) for clinical indicators, and by Dr Bill Taylor (chair, Fellowship by Assessment group, RCGP) and Fiona Dalziel (practice manager working part time for the Medical and Dental Defence Union of Scotland) for the organisational indicators. Dr Hunter led the patient experience discussions where Professor Roland had a conflict of interest as the supplier of one of the questionnaires. Professor Mike Pringle and Dr Brian McKinstry provided additional academic advice on the patient questionnaires.

None of the advisers had been involved in this type of political negotiation before, but they found that all sides were committed to the idea that quality could be measured (in part at least) and should be rewarded. However, the decisions taken were always those of the negotiating teams, and those discussions sometimes reflected significant differences between the sides, e.g., the importance given by the government side on the importance of improving access to GPs.

Past experience heavily influenced the discussions. For the clinical indicators, Dr Snell was influenced by a local scheme like QOF, which he had introduced into East Kent: the Primary Care Clinical Evaluation Project (PRICCE).[9] The organisational indicators were strongly influenced by the various RCGP schemes, such as the Quality Practice Award and Quality Team Development. Discussions about verification and inspection were informed by the Scottish experience of widespread practice visiting for practice accreditation (the Scottish equivalent of Quality Team Development).

The RCGP had traditionally not taken part in political negotiations: that was the role of the BMA, with the college leading on issues relating to quality of care. However, these negotiations were about quality of care. Despite this, the college decided to have no formal input into the process and avoided making public comments or statements. Nevertheless, the college had considerable indirect influence, partly because of the people present, some of whom had leading roles in the college, and partly because the organisational indicators were substantially drawn from college schemes.

The size and scope of the proposed quality framework was a regular issue for discussion. The NHS confederation started with the view that the framework should cover as many conditions as possible. This was based, in part, on Snell's experience of PRICCE. The GPC of the BMA shared the view that a comprehensive framework offered the best opportunity for substantial financial investment in general practice.

Despite the desire to include a broad range of clinical conditions, there remained important clinical areas where the advisers were unable to recommend satisfactory indicators. The most obvious of these were mental health and cancer. In these areas, it was easy to describe the characteristics of good care but hard to develop reliable and valid indicators that could be extracted from medical records. So, these areas remained distinctly under-represented. This gap was partially remedied by including cancer and mental health as required elements for significant event audit under the 'education and training' section of the organisational indicators.

EVIDENCE FOR QOF INDICATORS

For clinical indicators, the advisers generally used only established national guidelines and avoided developing new clinical guidance. This was difficult partly as there were four countries involved in the negotiation. For example, Scottish advice was not always the same as English advice, and English National Service Frameworks held no automatic sway in Scotland. In general, evidence from individual research papers was not included as a basis for indicators: the recommendation had to be based on a major national guideline or clear professional consensus.

Even where good evidence was available, it was not always possible to construct an appropriate indicator. For example, within the framework, there is an indicator relating to use of angiotensin-converting enzyme (ACE) inhibitors in heart failure. There was also evidence that beta blockers might have as great or possibly greater impact on mortality in heart failure than ACE inhibitors. An indicator on heart failure and beta blockers could logically have been included. However, national guidance was at that time couched in terms that included phrases such as 'should be started under the supervision of a specialist' or 'only start when heart failure is stable'. The academic advisers were not able to devise a safe indicator to reflect those concerns. Campbell and Lester further consider the challenges of operationalising suggested indicators in Chapter 3.

IT experts were included relatively late in the discussions. There were clearly going to be difficulties in extracting much of the data for the clinical indicators from GP computer systems. However, the advisers and negotiators started from the perspective that many countries in the world measure quality by using information that is used for billing. They saw this as an opportunity to develop IT systems in UK general practice that were designed to measure the quality of care. So, new computerised clinical (Read) codes had to be developed, and substantial changes were made to GP computer systems to accommodate this aim. To this day, electronic records in the United Kingdom remain the only large-scale system in the world designed around quality assessment and quality improvement. As it turned out, only a very small number of indicators could not be developed to allow data extraction from an electronic medical record.

Exception reporting was the subject of vigorous debate. The government side saw exception reporting as an opportunity for GPs to inappropriately exclude patients for personal financial gain. There was also concern that the most needy patients would be excluded in this way. The academic advisers thought that exception reporting was essential to get professional 'buy-in' to the framework.[10] Without exception reporting, GPs would have a financial incentive to give treatment that, in some cases, might be inappropriate or harmful.

For organisational indicators, the advisers used various existing quality improvement, mainly from the RCGP, as their starting point. At the start, there were more than 350 indicators considered; these were gradually reduced to a more manageable set. There was real difficulty in adopting indicators that had been designed for a voluntary quality-improvement scheme and putting them into a contractual framework with financial incentives. For example, indicators that ran along the lines of 'The practice has a policy on …' might work well as a part of quality-improvement scheme but would be too easily gamed as contractual indicators. How to avoid the risk of overt gaming was a regular discussion point.

To measure patient feedback, the government wanted a single national questionnaire so that groups of practices in primary care trusts (PCTs) and individual practices could be compared. The BMA preferred to give GPs a choice of questionnaires, a strategy that would prevent ready comparisons between GPs. The compromise agreed upon was to have two questionnaires, the general practice assessment questionnaire (GPAQ) and the improving practice questionnaire (IPQ). The negotiating teams were advised on the choice of questionnaires by independent academic referees. The BMA was understandably nervous about the introduction of questionnaires, knowing that they would not be popular with GPs. The outcome of the negotiations over questionnaires was a large reward for GPs for modest effort and no constraints on the way in which questionnaires were administered. This was seen as an intervention that would start to produce a cultural change encouraging

GPs to take more notice of the views of their patients. Since then, the use of patient questionnaires has indeed become commonplace in the NHS.

WEIGHTING INDICATORS FOR P4P

After the indicators had been selected, the advisers were asked to score them. They did this against an overall maximum of 1000 points, with no idea of what the total sum of money would be. Their job was to advise on the relative number of points for different areas and indicators, based on the estimated workload to achieve the care described. Expert advisers were asked to think of an 'average practice' and were given the mean prevalence of the various diseases in the United Kingdom. No information from the literature was given to guide the advisers in making these judgements. There was no suggestion that health gain should be a criterion for allocating points to indicators: this process was part of a pay negotiation, and workload for GPs was the sole criterion used to guide the judgements made.

Dr Hunter and Professor Roland first made their own initial judgements and then convened two small groups of GPs in Scotland and Manchester to repeat the exercise. (The English group also contained one practice manager.) The exercise therefore produced three sets of results for how the points should be distributed between the various indicators – one from the expert advisers, and one each from a Scottish and English group of GPs. There was a substantial degree of conformity, and based on the results, the expert advisers made recommendations on how the points should be allocated. The negotiating teams subsequently made some significant changes to the scores in the final version of QOF to reflect other factors that were judged important (e.g., policy priority given to an area).

The top and bottom levels for each indicator were also a subject for detailed discussion but ultimately were decided by the negotiating teams. Arguments were put forward that the availability of unlimited exception reporting should mean that the 'top' levels should be very high (95% or 100%), but, in general, lower percentages were chosen for the upper levels of achievement.

CONCLUSIONS

A number of features stand out from these developments. It was the first time that the BMA had taken part in detailed negotiations about quality of care on behalf of the profession. The negotiations were notable for taking place in a relatively informal atmosphere, where most of those involved in the discussion were practising GPs. Informed by evidence from the expert advisers, the discussions around what aspects of quality could be incentivised were like those one might expect in a practice trying to improve the quality of its care. The process for sifting evidence was unstructured and depended to a large degree on the academic advisers. The process has since become much more complex, more formal and more expensive.

The negotiations were unusual in that, for the first time, the BMA had engaged in detailed negotiations about the quality of general practice care. Quality had become a political issue, and the traditional divide between the BMA (politics and policy) and the RCGP (quality of care) became permanently blurred.

In many ways, therefore, the task of choosing indicators was much easier during these first negotiations than subsequently. The decision to base indicators on existing national guidelines or areas where there was clear professional consensus meant that few indicators were designed to lead to a change in widely accepted standards of clinical practice. The indicators were therefore less contentious than some that were introduced later, as the aim of the exercise had been to bring the standard of general practice up to widely accepted norms. The clinical indicators were therefore designed to be those that almost all doctors should be able to support. So, although GPs were concerned about the changes to practice that would be required in order to deliver on the new framework, criticism of the actual indicators was less marked than might have been expected for such a profound change in the way that GPs were paid.

REFERENCES

1. Wilson M. Report on 1986 LMC conference. *Br Med J*. 1986; **293**: 1384–6.
2. Baker R, Hearnshaw H, Cooper A, *et al*. Assessing the work of medical audit advisory groups in promoting audit in general practice. *Qual Health Care*. 1995; 4(4): 234–9.
3. Hearnshaw H, Baker R, Cooper A. A survey of audit activity in general practice. *Br J Gen Pract*. 1998; 48(427): 979–81.
4. Seddon ME, Marshall MN, Campbell SM, *et al*. Systematic review of quality of clinical care in general practice in the UK, Australia and New Zealand. *Qual Health Care*. 2001; **10**: 152–8.
5. Middleton E, Baker D. Comparison of social distribution of immunisation with measles, mumps and rubella vaccine, England, 1991-2001. *Br Med J*. 2003; **326**: 854.
6. Baker D, Middleton E. Cervical screening and health inequality in England in the 1990's. *J Epidemiol Community Health*. 2003; **57**: 417–23.
7. Department of Health. *A First Class Service: quality in the new NHS*. London: Department of Health; 1998.
8. Ibid.
9. Ibid.
10. Spooner A, Chapple A, Roland M. What makes British general practitioners take part in a quality improvement scheme? *J Health Serv Res Policy*. 2001; **6**: 145–50.

CHAPTER 3

Developing indicators and the concept of QOFability

Stephen Campbell and Helen Lester

SUMMARY

The Quality and Outcomes Framework (QOF) was described as world leading at its introduction.[1] This chapter describes how the scheme was further developed by primary care academic experts after its introduction. The main focus, however, is on the new process for developing clinical QOF indicators led by the National Institute for Health and Clinical Excellence (NICE). Clinical areas are now prioritised by a NICE-appointed advisory committee, which then undergo a formal consensus procedure, followed by piloting in representative practices across England. This chapter also describes the concept of 'QOFability', which is shorthand used by the authors to describe reasons why certain issues can or cannot be made into QOF indicators. These reasons include the prevalence of the clinical issue, the accuracy of data extraction from general practice clinical systems, the clarity of diagnosis, the relevance of incentivised actions, how directly change can be attributed to primary care staff and consideration of any possible unintended consequences of introducing the proposed indicator.

Lessons are drawn from the experiences of other countries in developing pay-for-performance schemes. The chapter concludes by recommending a renewed, consistent and transparent focus on creating feasible, valid, reliable and piloted 'QOFable' clinical indicators.

Key points
- Since its introduction in 2004, the QOF has gone through one major (2006) and one minor (2009) reorganisation.
- Between 2005 and 2009, new indicators were developed by a group of appointed primary care academic experts in each QOF area.

- The method of developing the QOF changed with the introduction of a new NICE-led process for developing and piloting QOF indicators in April 2009.
- There remain unresolved tensions at the heart of the QOF – is it a mechanism for paying GPs, rewarding the attainment of quality targets or a quality improvement tool?
- The concept of 'QOFability' relates to why certain issues can or cannot be made into QOF indicators.

INTRODUCTION

The Quality and Outcomes Framework (QOF) was introduced in the United Kingdom in April 2004 as part of a new General Medical Services (GMS) contract for primary care. It was, in essence, a product of the factors described in Chapter 2; there were no real standards for general practice from the 1950s with general practitioners (GPs) acting almost entirely on their own conscience.[2] However, by the late 1990s, this had 'changed utterly'[3] because of multiple policy drivers. In particular, public disquiet over the quality and safety of healthcare services, the rise of evidence-based medicine, a change in the culture of the profession to recognise variation in the quality of primary care and serious under-funding of primary healthcare in the United Kingdom compared with other countries were the key factors underpinning its introduction.[4] Importantly, when compared with the experiences of pay-for-performance (P4P) in other countries, the government, for the first time, was willing to invest up to 20% of the primary care budget, 90% of which was new money, to develop a series of incentivised evidence-based indicators in primary care. However, there remain unresolved tensions at the heart of the QOF – is it a mechanism for paying GPs, rewarding the attainment of quality targets or a quality improvement tool?

The QOF originally consisted of 146 indicators. While the majority of these indicators were focused on clinical areas, the use of a 'balanced score card' approach is reflected in the mixture of clinical, organisational and patient-focused elements to the framework (*see* Box 3.1). Points for individual indicators were awarded in relation to the level of achievement of that indicator (e.g., the percentage of people with diabetes as well as blood pressure below a defined target), with a graduated scale of payments that started above a minimum threshold (25% initially but raised to 40% in 2006) and ended once a maximum threshold (usually 90%) was reached.

Since 2004, the QOF has gone through one major (2006) and one minor (2009) reorganisation. In 2006, seven new clinical domains were added (depression, atrial fibrillation, chronic kidney disease, dementia, obesity, palliative care and learning disability), and the clinical points were increased to 655 (66% of the total points) within a slightly reduced overall framework of 1000 points. In 2009, the main changes were the addition of a new area of primary prevention for heart disease (making the clinical indicators worth 697 points or 70% of the framework).

> **Box 3.1** The original QOF (2004–06)
>
> - Clinical Domain:
>   Seventy-six indicators in 11 areas (coronary heart disease, left ventricular dysfunction, stroke and transient ischaemic attack, hypertension, diabetes mellitus, chronic obstructive pulmonary disease, epilepsy, hypothyroidism, cancer, mental health and asthma) worth up to a maximum of 550 points (52.4% of the total).
>
> - Organisational Domain:
>   Fifty-six indicators in five areas (records and information, patient communication, education and training, medicines management, clinical and practice management) worth up to 184 points (17.5% of the total).
>
> - Patient Experience Domain:
>   Four indicators in two areas (Patient Survey and Consultation Length) worth up to 100 points (9.5% of the total).
>
> - Additional Services Domain:
>   Ten indicators in four areas (cervical screening, child health surveillance, maternity services and contraceptive services) worth up to 36 points (3.4% of the total).
>
> - Depth of Quality Measures:
>   A holistic care payment measures achievement across the clinical domain and is worth up to 100 points (9.5% of the total). A quality practice payment measures overall achievement in the organisational, patient experience and additional services domains and is worth up to 30 points (2.9% of the total). A target level of achievement on patient access to clinical care (access bonus) is rewarded with 50 points (4.8% of the total).

Three new sexual health indicators were added to additional services, and changes were made to patient experience so that data were collected through a new national survey. Funding for the changes introduced since 2006 was largely released by the removal of a number of organisational indicators and reducing the depth of quality measures.

Although the QOF is a voluntary system, more than 99% of UK practices now participate. During the first year, the levels of achievement exceeded those anticipated by the government, with an average of 83.4% of the available incentive payments claimed.[5] Achievements have increased in subsequent years with a very slight fall in 2008/09, largely due to changes in the patient experience domain (www.ic.nhs. uk/webfiles/QOF/2008-09/QOF%20Achievement%20and%20Prevalence%20 Bulletin%202008-09.pdf).

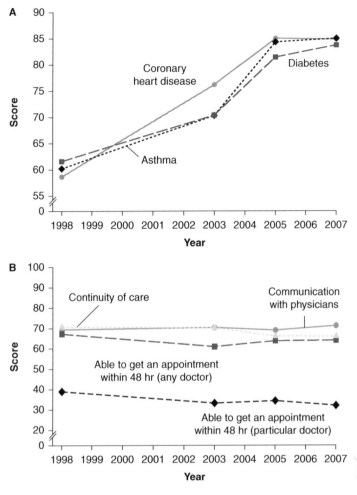

FIGURE 3.1 Mean scores for the quality of care at the practice level, 1998–2007

THE EXPERT PANEL PROCESS (2005–09)

From 2005 to 2009, new indicators were developed by a group of appointed primary care academics in each QOF clinical area (the Expert Panel), supported by a group of clinicians who also had an interest in that area. The topics for development came from two 'calls for evidence' in 2005 and 2007, which were widely distributed by primary care trusts, the British Medical Association (BMA), National Health Service (NHS) employers and voluntary groups such as the Long Term Conditions Alliance. More than 500 ideas regarding the topic areas were submitted from a wide range of stakeholders, including individuals, patient groups, professionals, charities, National Institute for Health and Clinical Excellence (NICE), the Department of Health and the pharmaceutical industry (who were asked to declare any financial interest in their submission) (*see* Figure 3.2).

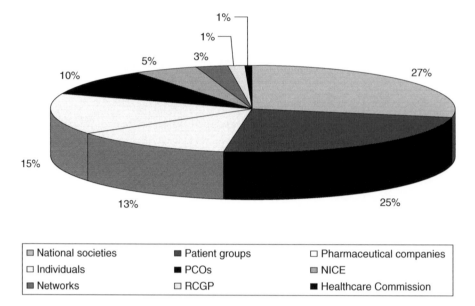

FIGURE 3.2 Range of groups submitting ideas in 2007 ($n = 153$)

These ideas were then prioritised by the Department of Health and General Practitioners Committee (GPC), and up-to-date evidence was reviewed in the selected areas. In 2007, two new elements were introduced into the development process. First, meetings were set up with 20 groups who had submitted prioritised ideas to ensure that the Expert Panel understood the intention behind the suggestions and also so as to explain to groups why some ideas were not suitable for inclusion in the QOF. This reflected a perception that, although some newspapers were interested in informing the public about the financial implications of the QOF[6] (and indeed most GPs received an increase in their earnings in the first year of the QOF of up to 25%), there was far less information available to the general public about the purpose of QOF or why only certain conditions were prioritised. Second, a modified Delphi Procedure[7] was included in the development process to combine available evidence with expert professional opinion. This enabled the development of indicators where evidence was patchy or inconclusive.[8]

Indicators were then commented on by a national patient organisation and general practice clinical systems experts in terms of their feasibility for implementation. The final set of published QOF indicators represented a negotiated compromise between the Department of Health, which needed to ensure the best possible use of treasury resources for patient benefit, and the BMA, representing the views and interests of the medical profession.

The new process under NICE

Since April 2009, NICE has led the process of developing the QOF. While it is not the aim of this chapter to describe this in detail, a series of important changes should improve the quality of future indicators. That NICE is an independent organisation means that political pressures to include particular topics or types of measure can be considered in a neutral manner. NICE also has a well-deserved reputation as a transparent organisation, with committees open to the public and relevant documents available on the web (www.nice.org.uk/aboutnice/qof/qof.jsp). This is reducing some of the previous mystique around the process of developing the QOF.

The process led by NICE focuses on developing clinical rather than other types of indicators. This reflects a trend that saw 52% of the framework related to clinical care in 2004, increasing to 66% on 2006 and 70% in 2009, respectively. Clinical areas and evidence-based statements within them are now prioritised by the 30 strong NICE-appointed advisory committee. These then go through a two-stage modified RAND appropriateness method[9] (which includes area experts and front-line GPs) where they are rated for their necessity.

Indicators are also reviewed at this early stage by specialists in general practice clinical systems, who can comment on feasibility, request Read codes and start to work on the underpinning business rules. Most importantly, the indicators that come through the consensus process (approximately 40%–50%) are now piloted in 30 representative practices across England and in a smaller number of practices in the devolved nations. This means that the final indicators presented to the Department of Health (DH)/GPC negotiators have been tested in real-world settings. In each pilot, the indicators will be tested for their data extraction feasibility and reliability across all general practice clinical systems. Data on the workload entailed will feed into the cost-effectiveness analysis of each indicator. In each pilot, qualitative interviews will be undertaken with general practice staff and patients to ask them their opinion of the value of each piloted indicator to place the opinions of staff and patients at the heart of the piloting process. This process is, however, time consuming, and the first indicators from the new NICE-led process will not become part of the QOF until at least April 2011. Indeed, the full benefits of the entire process will not become apparent until April 2012.

What makes a good QOF indicator? (QOFability)

Ideally, a QOF indicator – like any other quality indicator – should exhibit key characteristics, such as validity and sensitivity to change. Achievement against the indicator should be attributable directly to the actions of those being assessed (*see* Box 3.2).[10] However, there are a number of additional 'QOFability' hurdles that each potential area and indicator need to pass before they can be considered for potential introduction into the QOF. First, a clinical area has to be common but also important in terms of morbidity and, to some extent, mortality. For example, otitis media is extremely common, but significantly associated morbidity is relatively small, which means it is unlikely to ever become part of the QOF. Multiple sclerosis has very significant morbidity but is relatively rare. Although an average practice of 6300 patients might expect to have about eight people with multiple sclerosis on their list, a single-handed practice might only have one or two patients. Multiple sclerosis is therefore also unlikely to become part of the QOF.

Box 3.2 The ideal attributes of a quality indicator

- *Acceptability:* is acceptable to both those being assessed and those undertaking the assessment.

- *Attributable:* achievement of the aspect of care defined by an indicator should be 100% under the control of those being assessed.
  Fifty-six indicators in five areas (records and information, patient communication, education and training, medicines management, clinical and practice management) worth up to 184 points (17.5% of the total).

- *Feasibility:* valid, reliable and consistent data are available and collectable.

- *Reliability:* minimal measurement error, reproducible findings when administered by different raters (inter-rater reliability).

- *Sensitivity to change:* has the capacity to detect changes in quality of care, to discriminate between and within subject.

- *Predictive value:* has the capacity to predict quality of care outcomes.

- *Relevance:* be in an area where there is a recognised gap between actual and potential performance.

Each QOF domain also needs to be internally coherent, with indicators in a logical order. If only one or two elements of a potential suite of indicators can be made to work within the IT confines of the QOF, then there is less value in introducing the domain.

From a general practice clinical systems' perspective, indicators also need to be unambiguous, able to be extracted in a clear, sequential and consistent manner from a range of general practice computer systems through the central quality management and analysis system (QMAS). This partly accounts for why many QOF indicators are single disease and single issue in their focus.

Indicators within the QOF should also be evidence based rather than policy based. All submissions during the previous Expert Panel process needed to state clearly the evidence base underpinning the proposal, and almost all of the current QOF indicators are based on evidence from national guidance. In the new NICE-led process, all indicators are underpinned by NICE or Scottish Intercollegiate Guidelines Network (SIGN) guidance with an aspiration in 2010 to use NHS evidence (www.evidence.nhs.uk) as a source.

To be truly 'QOFable', a condition has to be something that can be clearly defined and diagnosed. For example, osteoarthritis of the knee is a common condition with significant morbidity that affects 12% of people above age 65.[11] Diagnosis can be difficult and is usually made on clinical grounds. There is potential for significant variation in prevalence and therefore general practice payments because of different GPs' subjective opinions on whether someone has osteoarthritis of the knee or not. The QOF could incentivise a referral for X-ray confirmation, but that has implications for secondary-care radiology services (*see* later) and conflicts with current radiology guidelines.[12] There are a number of conditions that might seem to be ideal candidates for the QOF at face value, but which fall at the fence of diagnostic ambiguity.

A condition, or indicator related to it, also has to be something that every primary care team in the land could address. An indicator that requires referral for a scan that is not uniformly available to every practice in the United Kingdom would not be 'QOFable'. This has been a problem when trying, for example, to develop an osteoporosis domain for the QOF. Osteoporosis is a prevalent condition with significant morbidity and mortality,[13] but access to bone density or dual energy X-ray absorptiometry (DEXA) scans is not yet universal. While not all osteoporosis indicators rely on DEXA scan results, this would be an early indicator in any potential domain. There is a counter argument that the QOF could drive service innovation and that therefore availability should not be included in a 'QOFability' debate. However, it is difficult to argue that the QOF should be used as a tool to improve secondary-care provision in a time of financial austerity and within a system of multiple funding streams.

Attribution to primary care further defines a good QOF indicator. While outcome measures are often seen as the 'gold standard', process measures are more useful as a measure of performance in primary care. Hard outcomes such as mortality or smoking cessation rates are, of course, influenced by primary care, but they often result long after that care has been given. They are influenced by patient lifestyle choices and socio-demographic factors outside the control of primary care staff as well as the availability of secondary-care services.[14] Casemix adjustment can, in theory, be used to adjust outcomes for underlying differences between populations.[15] However, there is usually insufficient information in the medical record to do this for practice populations. Intermediate outcome measures, linked to true outcomes based on scientific evidence, are the more useful indicators in primary care. The QOF has a number of such intermediate outcomes, e.g., those focused on lowering blood pressure in people with heart disease where there is evidence that controlling blood pressure improves survival.[16] However, they are more difficult to achieve and represent a greater workload, which is why they attract more points than simple process indicators and have lower achievement thresholds.

It is also important to be constantly mindful of unintended consequences of the QOF.[17] For example, we know that smoking is higher and cessation rates are lower in practices serving areas of higher deprivation.[18,19] If outcomes alone are prioritised, an indicator might relate to smoking cessation rates rather than referral for advice and treatment. This would affect practice income and could have the unintended consequence of dissuading GPs from practising in deprived areas, where health needs are greatest.[20]

The QOF indicators should focus on health inequalities and be cost-effective.[21] Although not originally designed as such, there is some evidence that the QOF is an equitable health intervention (*see* Chapters 5 and 6).[22] Cost-effectiveness is obviously important, particularly at a time of worldwide fiscal constraint, but, once again, it is important to note that nearly all QOF indicators are process-orientated, reflecting the work of primary care. They are not underpinned by a wealth of cost-effectiveness data (*see* www.york.ac.uk/inst/che/pdf/jointexecutivesummaryUEA-York-%20270308final.pdf (accessed 14 March 2010)).

The retirement of indicators that have reached their ceiling presents yet further challenges. De-selection requires rigorous analysis of achievement trends and exception reporting rates. Unwanted declines in achievement (as were seen when immunisation against influenza in patients with asthma was removed from the framework) may be mitigated by graduated reduction in payments.[23] QOFability issues are summarised in Box 3.3.

Lessons from and for other countries

The international evidence on P4P is discussed in Chapter 10, but it is interesting to compare and contrast how primary care P4P has been introduced in different countries. P4P schemes for primary care operate in Australia, New Zealand and the Netherlands.[24]

As described earlier, the UK QOF represents roughly 25% of a family doctor's income, and the QOF currently consists of 86 clinical indicators worth 697 points or nearly 70% of the framework. This contrasts sharply with the experience of using P4P in the United States. A national survey in the United States found that 52% of health management organisations (covering 81% of enrollees) reported using P4P.[25] Eighty per cent of rewards focused on clinical areas, matching closely to the current 2009 QOF. However, there was an average of only five performance measures per scheme. Rewards for reaching fixed thresholds dominated (62%)

Box 3.3 What makes an area or an indicator QOFable?

To be an ideal QOF indicator, the clinical issue in question should be:
- common
- have a significant morbidity and/or mortality
- lend itself to a series of logical and internally consistent indicators.

The indicator itself must be:
- extractable from QMAS in a non-ambiguous manner
- evidence based
- achievable by every primary care practice in the United Kingdom
- clearly defined
- attributable to actions in primary care
- free of obvious unintended consequences.

with only 23% rewarding improvement. The maximum bonus pay for physicians in the United States was 5%–10%. Therefore, in the United States, P4P is predominantly a payment mechanism for achieving fixed thresholds, with the proportion contributing to physician income substantially lower than the QOF in the United Kingdom. However, the primary purpose of incentivisation (through a payment mechanism or improvement scheme) is unclear in the United States. We would argue that too much money is currently attached to QOF in the United Kingdom, and that the evidence base in this area suggests that financial incentives are most likely to be effective in influencing professional behaviour when performance measures and rewards are aligned to the values of the staff being rewarded.[26] Indeed, external incentives may crowd out motivation – the desire to do a task well for its own sake – if they clash with the professional's perceptions of their role or identity and of quality care.[27] If measures and underlying data are not viewed as valid, physicians may see them as unfair or inappropriate.[28] One way forward is to reduce the overall size of the QOF and ensure that the indicators included are those that are most closely aligned to GPs' views of their role and the core work of primary care.

It is also important to consider P4P systems and quality indicators using intrinsic and/or contextual factors, as well as statistical or achievement rates. Contextual factors include the wider framework in which P4P is operating. For example, in the United Kingdom, before introduction of the QOF, there were data available on current baselines for quality of care within general practice.[29] Such baseline data are not available in most other countries. Data entry and extraction are key drivers in the way P4P can be and is being implemented. In the United Kingdom, the QOF operates using solely electronic data entry and extraction processes using agreed clinical (Read) codes. However, the level of computerised clinical information systems within general practices varies and is insufficient in Australia, Germany, New Zealand and the United States to use this method.[30] Moreover, the golden rule of the QOF in the United Kingdom is 'first, create a register'. This is only possible because patients register currently with only one GP and the QOF is a practice/team-based initiative. GPs in the United Kingdom also act as gatekeepers to specialist care. This is not the case in many other countries.[31] The method of payment for family practices/physicians is also important. In most countries, unlike, e.g., the United Kingdom or the Netherlands, this is largely based on fees-for-service, with patients paying a proportion of the fee. As discussed earlier, one of the key attributes of a quality indicator is that it is attributable directly to those being assessed. Where patients can access more than one practice, this has implications for payment mechanisms that reward the provision of services. As such, the introduction of P4P must take place within the context of the financial structures and regulatory systems in which primary care organisations work as well as linkages between sectors, the available skills of healthcare staff and baseline data for current quality of care. What should be or can be made QOFable in any country therefore depends on these characteristics of the host system.

CONCLUSIONS

The QOF, under NICE, is now developing in a more systematic and transparent manner – but there are plenty of challenges ahead. As the population demography changes, patients are increasingly likely to present with more than one condition.[32,33] Primary care will provide the majority of ongoing care for this growing population within most healthcare systems. There is therefore a need to develop, pilot and validate sets of measures that take into account the number and severity of conditions at an individual level.

There are unresolved tensions around the purpose of the QOF that continue to affect national negotiations. If the QOF is to be predominantly seen as a quality-improvement scheme rather than a payment mechanism, the focus should be on creating feasible, valid, reliable, 'QOFable' clinical indicators that are piloted, used and removed in an accepted manner.[34] They could also be aligned with other organisational and patient experience initiatives in a systems-based quality improvement strategy. If the United Kingdom succeeds with such an approach, it may finally lay claim to Paul Shekelle's description of the boldest initiative to improve the quality of primary care ever attempted in the world.[35]

REFERENCES

1. Shekelle P. New contract for general practitioners. *BMJ*. 2003; **326**: 457–8.
2. Collings JS. General practice in England today: a reconnaissance. *Lancet*. 1950; i; 555–85.
3. Smith R. All changed, utterly changed. *BMJ*. 1998; **316**: 1917–18.
4. Roland M. Linking physicians' pay to the quality of care—a major experiment in the United Kingdom. *New Engl J Med*. 2004; **351**: 1448–54.
5. Doran T, Fullwood C, Gravelle H, *et al*. Pay-for-performance programs in family practices in the United Kingdom. *New Engl J Med*. 2006; **355**: 375–84.
6. www.healthcarerepublic.com/GP/news/950496/Complaint-settled-media-coverage-GP-pay/ (accessed 21 December 2009).
7. Campbell SM, Braspenning J, Hutchinson A, *et al*. Research methods used when applying and developing quality indicators in primary care. *Qual Safe Health Care*. 2002; **11**: 358–64.
8. Jones JJ, Hunter D. Consensus methods for medical and health services research. *BMJ*. 1995; **311**: 376–80.
9. Campbell, Braspenning, Hutchinson, *et al.*, op. cit.
10. Ibid.
11. Brion PH, Kalunian KC. *Oxford Textbook of Medicine*. 4th ed. Sec. 18.8. Oxford: Oxford University Press; 2003.
12. National Institute for Health and Clinical Excellence. *Osteoarthritis Full Guidance*. London: NICE; 2008. www.nice.org.uk/nicemedia/pdf/CG059FullGuideline.pdf (accessed 13 December 2009).
13. SIGN. *Management of Osteoporosis. Guideline 71*. Edinburgh: SIGN; 2003.
14. Giuffrida A, Gravelle H, Roland M. Measuring quality with routine data: avoiding confusion between performance indicators and health outcomes. *BMJ*. 1999; **319**: 94–8.

15. Lilford RJ, Brown CA, Nicholl J. Use of process measures to monitor the quality of clinical practice. *BMJ.* 2007; **335**: 648–50.
16. Collins R, Peto R, McMahon S, *et al.* Blood pressure, stroke, and coronary artery disease. Part 2, short-term reductions in blood pressure: overview of randomized trials in their epidemiological context. *Lancet.* 1990; **335**: 827–38.
17. Roland M. The Quality and Outcomes Framework: too early for a final verdict. *Br J Gen Pract.* 2007; **57**: 525–7.
18. Layte R, Whelan CT. *Explaining Social Class Differentials in Smoking: The Role of Education. Working paper 12.* London: Economic and Social Research Institute; 2004.
19. Esteve F, Schiaffino A, Borrell C, *et al.* Social class, education, and smoking cessation: long-term follow-up of patients treated at a smoking cessation unit. *Nicotine Tobacco Res.* 2006; **8**(1): 29–36.
20. Tudor Hart J. The inverse care law. *Lancet.* 1971; **297**: 405–12.
21. National Institute for Health and Clinical Excellence. *Developing Clinical and Health Improvement Indicators for the Quality and Outcomes Framework (QOF) Interim Process Guide.* London: NICE; 2009. www.nice.org.uk/media/742/32/QOFProcessGuide.pdf (accessed 21 December 2009).
22. Doran T, Fullwood C, Kontopantelis E, *et al.* Effect of financial incentives on inequalities in the delivery of primary clinical care in England: analysis of clinical activity indicators for the Quality and Outcomes Framework. *Lancet.* 2008; **372**: 728–36.
23. Reeves D, Doran T, Valderas J, *et al.* How to identify when a performance indicator has run its course. *BMJ.* 2010; **340**: 899–901.
24. Schoen C, Osborn R, Trang Huynh R, *et al.* On the front lines of care: primary care doctors' office systems, experiences, and views in seven countries. *Health Aff.* 2006; **25**: w555–w571.
25. Rosenthal MB, Landon BE, Normand SL, *et al.* Pay for performance in commercial HMOs. *New Engl J Med.* 2006; **355**: 1895–902.
26. Marshall M, Smith P. Rewarding results: using financial incentives to improve quality. *Qual Safe Health Care.* 2003; **12**: 397–8.
27. Gagné M, Deci EL. Self-determination theory and work motivation. *J Org Behav.* 2005; **26**: 331–62.
28. Bokhour BG, Burgess JF, Hook J, *et al.* Incentive implementation in physician practices: a qualitative study of practice executive perspectives on pay for performance. *Med Care Res Rev.* 2006; **63**: 73s–95s.
29. Campbell SM, Steiner A, Robison J, *et al.* Is the quality of care in general medical practice improving? Results of a longitudinal observational study. *Br J Gen Pract.* 2003; **53**: 298–304.
30. Schoen, Osborn, Trang Huynh, *et al.*, op. cit.
31. Engels Y, Campbell SM, Dautzenberg M, *et al.* Developing a framework of, and quality indicators for, general practice management in Europe. *Fam Pract.* 2005; **22**: 215–22.
32. Berenson RA, Horvath J. Confronting the barriers to chronic care management in Medicare. *Health Aff.* 2003; Supplement web exclusives W3: 37–53.
33. Fortin M, Bravo G, Hudon C. Prevalence of multimorbidity among adults seen in family practice. *Ann Fam Med.* 2005; **3**: 223–8.
34. Reeves, Doran, Valderas, *et al.*, op. cit.
35. Shekelle, op. cit.

Impact of the Quality and Outcomes Framework

CHAPTER 4

Learning from the QOF: a review of existing research

Nicholas Steel and Sara Willems

SUMMARY

This chapter reviews the evidence about the effects of the Quality and Outcomes Framework (QOF) on healthcare, including unintended outcomes and equity. Relevant papers were identified by searching the MEDLINE database and from the reference lists of published reviews and papers. A separate systematic literature review was conducted to identify papers with information on the impact of the framework on inequalities. All studies were observational, and so it cannot be assumed that any changes were caused by the framework. The results both for individual indicators and from different studies vary substantially. The diverse nature of the research precluded formal synthesis of data from different studies. Achievement of quality standards was high when the contract was introduced and has risen each year roughly in line with the pre-existing trend. Inequalities in achievement of standards were generally small when the framework was implemented, and most have reduced further since. There is weak evidence that achievement for conditions outside the framework was lower initially and has neither worsened nor improved since the QOF was introduced. Some interventions in the framework may be cost-effective. Professionals feel consultations and continuity have suffered to some extent. There is very little research about patients' views or about the aspects of general practice not measured, such as caring, context and complexity. The chapter concludes that the evidence base about the impact of the QOF is growing but remains patchy and inconclusive. More high-quality research is needed to inform decisions about how the framework should change to maximise improvements in health and equity.

Key points

- UK primary care practices have received substantial financial rewards for achievement of quality standards set out in the QOF.
- National reported achievement of clinical quality standards by practices for payment was generally high at baseline and has risen each year since.
- This chapter reports on the published evidence about the effects of the QOF.
- Findings come from observational studies and vary between indicators and studies.
- Achievement of standards has risen each year by approximately the amount that would have been expected from continuation of the trend that existed before April 2004, with no consensus that the introduction of the framework altered the underlying overall rate of quality improvement.
- There is some weak evidence of cost effectiveness and increasing equity, again with variability between studies and between indicators.
- Consultations and continuity of care may have been affected.
- There is very little research into patients' views or the aspects of general practice not measured by the framework.

INTRODUCTION

Many people still do not receive healthcare that has been shown to improve outcomes, even when healthcare systems are well funded and widely available.[1,2] As we have seen, the Quality and Outcomes Framework (QOF) rewards achievement of standards in four domains: clinical, organisational, additional services and patient experience (*see* Box 4.1).[3] The clinical domain initially contained standards for 10 chronic conditions, rising to 20 in 2009/10.[4]

The scale of reward payments is far greater than previous performance-related payments to UK general practices for immunisations, cervical screening or health promotion clinics. The new contract was described as a 'radical experiment'.[6] It was an experiment on a very large scale, without a comparison group and with no planned evaluation, and so the rapidly growing numbers of publications about the effects of the contract rely on observational evidence, and innovative use of existing datasets.

Pay-for-performance (P4P), or payment for quality, is now part of the health policy landscape in many countries, and there is widespread interest in the extent to which it can change outcomes.[7,8] In the United Kingdom, the QOF continues to evolve and is likely to become increasingly evidence based under the stewardship of the National Institute for Health and Clinical Excellence (NICE).[9] This chapter sets out to review the published research evidence about the effects of the QOF in the United Kingdom on healthcare processes and outcomes,[10] including unintended outcomes, e.g., effects on unincentivised care and equity in healthcare.

Box 4.1 Domains for quality indicators in the QOF 2009[5]

Clinical domain
  Secondary prevention of coronary heart disease
  Cardiovascular disease: primary prevention
  Heart failure
  Stroke and transient ischaemic attack
  Hypertension
  Diabetes mellitus
  Chronic obstructive pulmonary disease
  Epilepsy
  Hypothyroid
  Cancer
  Palliative care
  Mental health
  Asthma
  Dementia
  Depression
  Chronic kidney disease
  Atrial fibrillation
  Obesity
  Learning disabilities
  Smoking

Organisational domain
  Records and information
  Information for patients
  Education and training
  Practice management
  Medicines management

Patient experience domain
  Length of consultations
  Patient survey (access)

Additional services
  Cervical screening
  Child health surveillance
  Maternity services
  Contraception

Search strategy

This review is limited to the QOF; the wider literature on P4P is considered in Chapter 10. Included papers relevant to the QOF were identified from the reference lists of two recent reviews of the international literature on P4P,[11,12,13] as well as from other published papers and authors in the field. A supplementary electronic literature search for more recent papers (up to 26 January 2010) was conducted using MEDLINE. To study the impact of the QOF on inequalities, a separate systematic literature review was conducted using MEDLINE, Embase, the Cochrane Library, Web of Science, PsychInfo and Econlit. Studies with a longitudinal or serial cross-sectional design were included, and the quality of the selected studies was appraised based on the criteria of the Dutch Cochrane Centre.

RESULTS

Most research into the effects of the QOF has concentrated on the clinical domain. Twenty-nine studies examined the impact of the QOF on healthcare, four reported on the impact on professionals and two reported on costs (*see* Table 4.1). Nearly all relevant studies were observational studies, cross-sectional, repeated cross-sectional (before and after contract implementation) or cohort studies. Most data had been collected after contract implementation in 2004, but some studies included pre-QOF data.

Achievement of quality indicators

Analysis of QOF data from all general practices in England showed that the median overall achievement reported by practices was high in year 1 (85.1%; interquartile range, 79.0–89.1) and increased to 89.3% in year 2 and 90.8% in year 3.[43,44] A median of 5.3% of patients were excluded by practices from their returns, as being unsuitable for the indicator.[45]

Diabetes is the most studied QOF condition. National QOF data show substantial improvements in diabetes care from 2004 to 2008, with the percentage of 'low-performing' practices dropping from 57% to 26%.[46] A systematic review found that the quality of care reported in the QOF was higher than that in previously published studies,[47] and improvements in quality in diabetes have been consistently found in studies that used either QOF or non-QOF data. Diabetes care in Scotland improved from 2004 to 2005[48]; the Wandsworth Prospective Diabetes Study found improved support for smoking cessation in those with diabetes from 2003 to 2005[49]; improvements in performance ranged from 6.6% to 42.8% in general practices in North Warwickshire from 2004 to 2005,[50] and from 9.2% to 40.9% in Shropshire from 2004 to 2006.[51,52] One small hospital-based study reported an increase in referrals for poor glycaemic control.[53]

TABLE 4.1 Impact of the QOF on health outcomes: description of studies reviewed

First author and paper	Condition	Study time period	Design	Data source	Sample size and setting	Results
Doran (2006): Pay-for-performance programs in family practices in the United Kingdom.[14]	Multiple: 10 conditions	2004–05	Cross-sectional survey	National Health Service (NHS) quality management and analysis system (QMAS)	8105 general practices in England	Median of 96.7% of the available points for clinical indicators. (Asthma, cancer, CHD, chronic obstructive airways disease, diabetes mellitus, epilepsy, hypertension, hypothyroidism, severe mental health and stroke)
Doran (2008): Exclusion of patients from pay-for-performance targets by English physicians.[15]	Multiple: 10 conditions	2005–06	Cross-sectional survey	NHS QMAS	8105 general practices in England	Median of 5.3% of patients excluded [interquartile range (IQR): 4.0–6.9]. (Asthma, cancer, CHD, chronic obstructive airways disease, diabetes mellitus, epilepsy, hypertension, hypothyroidism, severe mental health and stroke)
Doran (2008): Effect of financial incentives on inequalities in the delivery of primary clinical care in England: analysis of clinical activity indicators for the Quality and Outcomes Framework.[16]	Multiple: 11 conditions	2004–07	Retrospective longitudinal survey	NHS QMAS	7637 general practices in England	Median overall reported achievement was 85.1% (IQR: 79.0–89.1) in year 1, 89.3% (86.0–91.5) in year 2 and 90.8% (88.5–92.6) in year 3. (Asthma, cancer, CHD, heart failure, chronic obstructive airways disease, diabetes mellitus, epilepsy, hypertension, hypothyroidism, severe mental health and stroke)

(Continued)

TABLE 4.1 Impact of the QOF on health outcomes: description of studies reviewed (Continued)

First author and paper	Condition	Study time period	Design	Data source	Sample size and setting	Results
Fleetcroft (2008): Potential population health gain of the Quality and Outcomes Framework. In: *Quality and Outcomes Framework. Joint executive summary: Reports to the Department of Health.*[17]	Multiple: 10 conditions	2004–06	Modelling study	Literature review	Literature review	In the 2003 General Medical Services (GMS) contract the potential lives saved per 100 000 populations per year aggregated at the domain level are: 163.2 lives in CHD, 109.5 lives in diabetes, 53.6 lives in hypertension, 44.9 lives in stroke, 27.6 lives in chronic obstructive pulmonary disease, 11.6 lives in left ventricular dysfunction and 8.8 lives in asthma. There was potential for 415.77 lives saved per 100 000 per year (400.32–444.99) aggregated across all clinical indicators and domains
MacBride-Stewart (2008): Do quality incentives change prescribing patterns in primary care? An observational study in Scotland.[18]	Multiple: eight conditions	2002–06	Retrospective observational study	Prescribing Information System for Scotland	92 practices in Lothian Scotland	The prescribing of QOF drugs increased significantly faster than the non-QOF drugs both before and after the introduction of the latest GMS contract but the rate of increase for the QOF drugs slowed significantly after April 2005 unlike prescribing of non-QOF drugs. Increases in prescribing per month for QOF and non-QOF drugs during the

Reference	Condition	Year	Study design	Data source	Practices	Findings
Downing (2007): Do the government's new Quality and Outcomes Framework (QOF) scores adequately measure primary care performance? A cross sectional survey of routine healthcare data.[19]	Multiple: six conditions	2004–05	Ecological cross-sectional study	QOF data, emergency hospital admissions and all cause mortality	All general practices in two English Primary Care Trusts	2-year periods before and after April 2005. QOF 1.32 before, 1.01 after, $p < 0.001$. Non-QOF 0.23 before, 0.32 after, $p = 0.09$. (CHD, heart failure, stroke, hypertension, diabetes mellitus, chronic obstructive airways disease, epilepsy and asthma) The associations between QOF scores and emergency admissions and mortality were small and inconsistent. (Asthma, cancer, chronic obstructive pulmonary disease, CHD, diabetes, stroke and 'all other conditions')
Hippisley-Cox (2007): Final report for the information centre for health and social care: time series analysis for 2001–2006 for selected clinical indicators from the Quality and Outcomes Framework.[20]	Multiple: six conditions	2001–06	Longitudinal cross-sectional survey	QRESEARCH database	498 general practices in England	There was an increase in the percentage achievement of all the quality indicators. Range of absolute increase in achievement of quality indicators in each condition: CHD: 28.3–42.1%, stroke: 33.8–47.9%, diabetes mellitus: 4.1–42.0%, epilepsy: 68.8% (only one quality improvement), hypertension: 15.7–28.5%, chronic kidney disease: 16.1–38.4%. (CHD,

(Continued)

TABLE 4.1 Impact of the QOF on health outcomes: description of studies reviewed (Continued)

First author and paper	Condition	Study time period	Design	Data source	Sample size and setting	Results
						stroke, diabetes mellitus, epilepsy, hypertension and chronic kidney disease)
Campbell (2007): Quality of primary care in England with the introduction of pay-for-performance.[21]	Multiple: three conditions	1998–2005	Longitudinal cohort study	Primary data collection	42 general practices in England	Difference between 2005 observed score and mean predicted score for 2005 on basis of 1998–03 trend: CHD 4.3%, diabetes 8.2%, asthma 12%. Mean difference between transformed observed score and predicted score for 2005: CHD 0.22% [95% confidence interval (CI) –0.02 to 0.45], diabetes 0.68 (0.27–1.1), asthma 0.44 (0.27–0.62). (CHD, asthma and diabetes)
Steel (2007): Quality of clinical primary care and targeted incentive payments: an observational study.[22]	Multiple: four conditions (two in QOF and two not in QOF)	2003–05	Retrospective observational cross-sectional study	Primary data collection	18 general practices in England	A significant increase occurred for the six indicators linked to incentive payments: from 75% achieved in 2003 to 91% in 2005 (change = 16%, 95% CI: 10–22%, $p < 0.01$). A significant increase also occurred for 15 other indicators linked to 'incentivised conditions'; 53–64% (change = 11%, 95% CI: 6–15%, $p < 0.01$). The 'non-incentivised conditions' started at a lower

						achievement level, and did not increase significantly: 35–36% (change = 2%, 95% CI: −1 to 4%, $p = 0.19$). (Asthma, hypertension, depression and osteoarthritis)
Gulliford (2007): Achievement of metabolic targets for diabetes by English primary care practices under a new system of incentives.[23]	Diabetes	Retrospective cohort study	Primary data collection	2000–05	26 practices in South London	Proportion of patients achieving HbA1c ≤7.4% each year increased: 2000, 22%; 2001, 32%; 2002, 37%; 2003, 38% and in 2005 from QOF, 57%
Khunti (2007): Quality of diabetes care in the UK: comparison of published quality-of-care reports with results of the Quality and Outcomes Framework for diabetes.[24]	Diabetes	Systematic review	Published observational studies of quality of diabetes care in primary care in the United Kingdom	1999–2006	Six studies	Improvement in both process and outcome of care. The quality of care reported in QOF was greater than that found in other published studies
Calvert (2009): Effect of the Quality and Outcomes Framework on diabetes care in the United Kingdom: retrospective cohort study.[25]	Diabetes	Retrospective cohort study	Doctors' independent network-LINK (from iSOFT, previously TOREX) age-sex similar	2002–07	147 UK general practices	Significant improvements in process and intermediate outcome measures were observed during the 6-year period, with consecutive annual improvements observed before the introduction of incentives.

(Continued)

TABLE 4.1 Impact of the QOF on health outcomes: description of studies reviewed (Continued)

First author and paper	Condition	Study time period	Design	Data source	Sample size and setting	Results
				to United Kingdom but practices in the south of England and higher socio-economic groups are over-represented		After the introduction of the QOF, existing trends of improvement in glycaemic control, cholesterol levels and blood pressure were attenuated
Srirangalingam (2006): Changing pattern of referral to a diabetes clinic following implementation of the new UK GP Contract.[26]	Diabetes	2003–04	Serial cross-sectional study (before and after)	Primary data collection	Referrals to Barts and The London NHS Trust	Increase in referrals for poor glycaemic control, and the glycaemic threshold for referral with poor glycaemic control has reduced [9.7% vs. 10.6%, $p =$ 0.006, mean difference = 0.9% (95% CI: 0.4–1.3%)]
Millett (2007): Impact of a pay-for-performance incentive on support for smoking cessation and on smoking prevalence among people with diabetes.[27]	Diabetes	2003–05	Longitudinal cross-sectional survey	Wandsworth Prospective Diabetes Study	32 general practices in Wandsworth	Significantly more patients with diabetes had their smoking status ever recorded in 2005 than in 2003 (98.8% vs. 90.0%, $p < 0.001$). The proportion of patients with documented smoking cessation advice also increased significantly over this period, from 48.0% to

Reference	Condition	Year	Study design	Data source	Setting	Results
Jaiveer (2006): Improvements in clinical diabetes care in the first year of the new General Medical Services contract in the UK.[28]	Diabetes	2004–05	Longitudinal cross-sectional survey	Primary data collection	13 practices in North Warwickshire	83.5% ($p < 0.001$). The prevalence of smoking decreased significantly from 20.0% to 16.2% ($p < 0.001$). Diabetes indicator performance improved range from 6.6% to 42.8% over time
McGovern (2008): Introduction of a new incentive and target-based contract for family physicians in the UK: good for older patients with diabetes but less good for women?[29]	Diabetes	2004–05	Serial cross-sectional study	Scottish Programme for Improving Clinical Effectiveness (SPICE)	310 general practices in Scotland	54.2% relative increase in the number of patients recorded as having diabetes. Measurement of HbA1c, blood pressure, serum creatinine and cholesterol significantly increased ($p < 0.05$)
Millett (2009): Pay-for-performance and the quality of diabetes management in individuals with and without comorbid medical conditions.[30]	Diabetes	1997–2005	Cohort study	General Practice Research Database	422 general practices	The percentage of diabetes patients with co-morbidity reaching blood pressure and cholesterol targets exceeded that predicted by the underlying trend during the first 2 years of P4P [by 3.1% (95% CI: 1.1–5.1) for BP and 4.1% (95% CI: 2.2–6.0) for cholesterol among patients with ≥5 co-morbidities in 2005]. The percentage

(Continued)

TABLE 4.1 Impact of the QOF on health outcomes: description of studies reviewed (Continued)

First author and paper	Condition	Study time period	Design	Data source	Sample size and setting	Results
						of patients meeting the HbA1c target in the first 2 years of this program was significantly lower than predicted by the underlying trend in all patients, with the greatest shortfall in patients without co-morbidity [3.8% (95% CI: 2.6–5.0) lower in 2005]
Tahrani (2007): Diabetes care and the new GMS contract: the evidence for a whole county.[31]	Diabetes	2004–06	Observational retrospective cross-sectional study	National Diabetes Audit and QOF data from Shropshire PCTs	66 practices in Shropshire	Significant improvements in the percentage of patients achieving targets for all quality indicators ($p < 0.001$). Range 9.2–40.9 [lower and upper CI for different indicators]
Tahrani (2008): Impact of practice size on delivery of diabetes care before and after the Quality and Outcomes Framework implementation.[32]	Diabetes	2004–06	Observational retrospective cross-sectional study	National Diabetes Audit and QOF data from Shropshire PCTs	66 practices in Shropshire	All quality indicators showed significant improvement following the QOF. Significant improvement in achieving glycaemic control targets following QOF implementation in both large and small practices ($p < 0.001$ for HbA1c ≤7.4% and 10%)

Study	Disease	Years	Study type	Data source	Setting	Findings
Vaghela (2008): Population intermediate outcomes of diabetes under pay-for-performance incentives in England from 2004 to 2008.[33]	Diabetes	2004–08	Longitudinal cross-sectional survey	QOF data from Information Centre for Health and Social Care	8192–8423 general practices in England	A1C target at the median practice increased from 59.1% (IQR: 51.7–65.9) in 2004–2005 to 66.7% (IQR: 60.6–72.7) in 2007–2008, blood pressure from 70.9% in 2004–2005 to 80.2% in 2007–2008, and cholesterol from 72.6% in 2004–2005 to 83.6% in 2007–2008. In 2004–2005, 57% of practices were low performing (range by region 42.4–69.9). In 2007–2008, 26% of practices were low performing (range 11.6–37.5)
Bottle (2007): Association between quality of primary care and hospitalization for coronary heart disease in England: national cross sectional study.[34]	CHD	2003, 2004 and 2005	Ecological cross-sectional study	QOF, hospital admissions and census data	All 303 primary care trusts in England	No significant association between the quality of CHD care, as measured by the QOF, and rates of elective or unplanned hospital admission for CHD by primary care trust in England
McGovern (2008): The effect of the UK incentive-based contract on the management of patients with coronary heart disease in primary care.[35]	CHD	2004–05	Serial cross-sectional study	SPICE	310 general practices in Scotland	Recording and prescribing increased by mean 17.1% after the introduction of the nGMS contract

(Continued)

TABLE 4.1 Impact of the QOF on health outcomes: description of studies reviewed (Continued)

First author and paper	Condition	Study time period	Design	Data source	Sample size and setting	Results
Williams (2006): Does a higher 'quality points' score mean better care in stroke? An audit of general practice medical records.[36]	Stroke	November 2004	Cross-sectional survey	Primary data collection from practice records	Two general practices, one in southwest London and one in Surrey	Higher QOF quality points did not reflect better adherence to RCP guidance. There remains considerable scope for improvement in computer data quality before they can be used to measure adherence to best practice
Simpson (2006): Effect of the UK incentive-based contract on the management of patients with stroke in primary care.[37]	Stroke or transient ischemic attack	2004–05	Serial cross-sectional study	SPICE	310 general practices in Scotland	Documentation of quality indicators increased over time, with absolute increases for individual indicators ranging from 1.3% to 52.1%
McElduff (2004): Will changes in primary care improve health outcomes? Modelling the impact of financial incentives introduced to improve quality of care in the UK.[38]	Cardiovascular disease	2003	Modelling study	Literature review	England and Wales	The greatest health gain in those aged 45–84 years would come from reaching cholesterol reduction targets. This could prevent 15 events per 10 000 per 5 years in people with CHD, seven events in those with a history of stroke, and seven events in those with diabetes. Achieving blood pressure control targets in hypertensive patients without the above conditions could prevent 15 cardiovascular

						events. Achieving other targets would have smaller impacts because high levels of care are already being achieved or because of the low prevalence of conditions or associated event risk
Ashworth (2008): Effect of social deprivation on blood pressure monitoring and control in England: a survey of data from the Quality and Outcomes Framework.[39]	Blood pressure	2005–07	Retrospective longitudinal survey	QOF data	8515 general practices in England	In 2005, 82.3% of adults (n = 52.8 million) had an up-to-date blood pressure recording; by 2007, this proportion had risen to 88.3% (n = 53.2 m)
Shohet (2007): The association between the quality of epilepsy management in primary care, general practice population deprivation status and epilepsy related emergency hospitalisations.[40]	Epilepsy	2004–05	Ecological cross-sectional study	QOF data from the NHS Information Centre and HES data	General practices and hospitals in the three counties of Norfolk, Suffolk and Cambridgeshire	Relatively strong and statistically significant relationship between the proportions of epilepsy-treated patients who are declared as seizure-free and the proportion of patients with an epilepsy-related emergency hospitalisation. In other words, the quality of care as incentivised by the QOF system appears to lead to improved outcomes in terms of minimising epilepsy-related emergency hospitalisation

(Continued)

TABLE 4.1 Impact of the QOF on health outcomes: description of studies reviewed (Continued)

First author and paper	Condition	Study time period	Design	Data source	Sample size and setting	Results
Coleman (2007): Impact of contractual financial incentives on the ascertainment and management of smoking in primary care.[41]	Smoking	1990–2005	Retrospective longitudinal survey	The Health Improvement Network	10.8 million patients in UK general practices in 1990 rising to 1.6 million in 2004	Compared with the first quarter of 2003, there was an increase up to the first quarter of 2004 in recording of smoking status [rate ratio (RR): 1.88, 95% CI: 1.87–1.89] and in brief advice to smokers (RR: 3.03, 95% CI: 2.98–3.09), which was sustained until the first quarter of 2005
Strong (2009): The UK Quality and Outcomes Framework pay-for-performance scheme and spirometry: rewarding quality or just quantity? A cross-sectional study in Rotherham, UK.[42]	Chronic obstructive pulmonary disease (COPD)				38 general practices in Rotherham	Spirometry as assessed by clinical records was to british thoracic society (BTS) standards in 31% of cases (range at practice level 0–74%). The categorisation of airflow obstruction according to the most recent spirometry results did not agree well with the clinical categorisation of COPD recorded in the notes (Cohen's kappa = 0.34, 0.30–0.38). Twelve per cent of patients on COPD registers had fev1 (% predicted) results recorded that did not support the diagnosis of COPD. There was no association between quality, as measured by adherence to BTS spirometry standards, and either QOF COPD9 achievement (Spearman's rho = −0.11), or QOF COPD10 achievement (rho = 0.01)

Improvements have also been reported for other conditions after the introduction of the contract, using both QOF and alternative data sources. Care for coronary heart disease (CHD), stroke and transient ischaemic attacks (TIAs), blood pressure and smoking indicators all improved.[54,55,56,57]

Underlying trends in quality

The improvements described earlier in recording of care after the introduction of the contract may, of course, have happened anyway – with or without the QOF. A number of studies have looked at underlying trends in quality of care in an attempt to estimate the effect of the new contract on existing trends. Several conditions had been the subject of major quality improvement initiatives before the QOF (*see* Discussion) and it would be reasonable to expect a background of improving quality in these conditions.

Data from nearly 500 English practices in QRESEARCH for 19 QOF indicators from 2001 to 2006 showed that the percentage achievement of these indicators improved in all ages and among men and women. In nearly all cases, the trend showed a gradual improvement over the 5 years, with little change around 2004.[58] The exceptions to this were for recorded blood pressure below 150/90 mmHg, recorded cholesterol below 5 mmol/L or blood pressure below 150/90 in those with stroke and blood pressure below 140/85 in those with chronic kidney disease, all of which appeared to show a slight increased improvement from around 2004, greater than the underlying trend. There was also a dramatic improvement in the percentage of those with epilepsy reported free of convulsions, but the report's authors comment that: 'the READ codes to record this [epilepsy indicator] were not in general use in general practice prior to April 2003 and so the increase is likely to represent an increase in recording rather than a true increase'.

A cohort study in 42 English general practices measured care for asthma, CHD and diabetes in 1998, 2003 and 2005, and compared 2005 care with that predicted on the basis of the 1998–2003 trend.[59] A small significant increase in measures was found for diabetes and asthma above the trend, but no significant difference for CHD. This is consistent with a retrospective cohort study of diabetes care in 26 practices in London, which found that the proportion of those with well-controlled diabetes (HbA1c, <7.4%) had increased each year from 2000 to 2005, and that the 2005 increase was the largest.[60]

A study of diabetes care in 422 general practices in the General Practice Research Database found that achievement of HbA1c targets was slightly lower than predicted by the underlying trend, while achievement of blood pressure and cholesterol targets was slightly higher.[61] A retrospective cohort study of 147 practices found that outcomes for diabetes care (glycaemic control, cholesterol levels and blood pressure) improved steadily from 2002 to 2005, and improvement was then attenuated between 2005 and 2007.[62]

TABLE 4.2 Impact of the QOF on professionals: description of studies reviewed

First author and paper	Condition	Study time period	Design	Data source	Sample size and setting	Results
Campbell (2008): The experience of pay-for-performance in English family practice: a qualitative study.[85]	Family physicians' and nurses' beliefs and concerns	2007	Qualitative semi-structured interview study.	Primary data collection	22 general practices across England	The findings suggest that it is not necessary to align targets to professional priorities and values to obtain behaviour change, although doing so enhances enthusiasm and understanding. It also led to unintended effects, such as the emergence of a dual QOF–patient agenda within consultations, potential deskilling of doctors as a result of the enhanced role for nurses in managing long-term conditions, a decline in personal/relational continuity of care between doctors and patients, resentment by team members not benefiting financially from payments, and concerns about an ongoing culture of performance monitoring in the United Kingdom
Maisey (2008): Effects of payment for performance in primary care: qualitative interview study.[86]	Professional roles and the delivery of primary care	2006	Qualitative semi-structured interview study	Primary data collection	12 general practices in eastern England	Improvements in teamwork and in the organisation, consistency and recording of care for conditions incentivised in the scheme, but not for non-incentivised conditions. Changed emphasis from 'patient led' consultations and listening to

McDonald (2007): Impact of financial incentives on clinical autonomy and internal motivation in primary care: ethnographic study.[87]	2004 (after introduction of contract)	Ethnographic case study	Primary data collection	Two English general practices	Practice organisation, clinical autonomy and internal motivation of doctors and nurses	Increase in the use of templates to collect data on quality of care. Implementation of financial incentives for quality of care did not seem to have damaged the internal motivation of the general practitioners studied, although more concern was expressed by nurses patients' concerns. Loss of continuity of care and of patient choice. Nurses experienced increased workload but enjoyed more autonomy and job satisfaction. Doctors acknowledged improved disease management and teamwork but expressed unease about 'box-ticking' and increased demands of team supervision, despite better terms and conditions. Doctors were less motivated to achieve performance indicators where they disputed the evidence on which they were based

(Continued)

TABLE 4.2 Impact of the QOF on professionals: description of studies reviewed (Continued)

First author and paper	Condition	Study time period	Design	Data source	Sample size and setting	Results
McGregor (2008): Impact of the 2004 GMS contract on practice nurses: a qualitative study.[88]	Practice nurses, perceptions of the changes in their work	2006	Qualitative interview study	Primary data collection	Practice nurses employed in general practices within NHS Greater Glasgow	Practice nurses were positive about the development of their professional role but had had mixed views about whether their status had changed. Most felt under-rewarded, irrespective of practice QOF achievement. All reported a substantial increase in workload, related to incentivised QOF domains with greater 'box-ticking' and data entry, and less time to spend with patients. Although the structure created by the new contract was generally welcomed, many were unconvinced that it improved patient care and felt other important areas of care were neglected. Concern was also expressed about a negative effect of the QOF on holistic care, including ethical concerns and detrimental effects on the patient–nurse relationship, which were regarded as a core value

TABLE 4.3 Impact of the QOF on costs: description of studies reviewed

First author and paper	Condition	Study time period	Design	Data source	Sample size and setting	Results
Mason (2008): The GMS Quality and Outcomes Framework: are the Quality and Outcomes Framework (QOF) indicators a cost effective use of NHS resources? In: *Quality and Outcomes Framework. Joint executive summary: Reports to the Department of Health*.[91]	Multiple: 12 conditions	2007	Cost effectiveness	Literature review		Cost effectiveness evidence for 12 indicators in the 2006 revised contract. The three most cost-effective indicators were using angiotensin-converting enzyme inhibitors or angiotensin receptor blockers for chronic kidney disease, anti-coagulant therapy for atrial fibrillation and beta-blockers for CHD. The per-patient payment in 2004–05 ranged from £0.13 (for a chronic kidney disease indicator) to £87.79 (for a mental health indicator). The cost effectiveness of an indicator varied by its baseline achievement
Fleetcroft (2006): Do the incentive payments in the new NHS contract for primary care reflect likely population health gains?[92]	Multiple: seven conditions	2004–05	Cost consequence	Literature review		Maximum payments for the eight preventive interventions examined make up 57% of the total maximum payment for all clinical interventions in the QOF. There appears to be no relationship between pay and health gain across these eight interventions

TABLE 4.4 Impact of the QOF on equity: description of studies reviewed

First author and paper	Condition	Study time period	Design	Data source	Sample size and setting	Results
Doran (2008): Effect of financial incentives on inequalities in the delivery of primary clinical care in England: analysis of clinical activity indicators for the Quality and Outcomes Framework.[108]	Multiple: 11 conditions	2004–07	Retrospective longitudinal survey	NHS QMAS	7637 general practices in England	In year 1, area deprivation was associated with lower levels of achievement, with median achievement ranging from 86.8% (82.2–89.6) for quintile 1 (least deprived) to 82.8% (75.2–87.8) for quintile 5 (most deprived). Betw een years 1 and 3, median achievement increased by 4.4% for quintile 1 and by 7.6% for quintile 5, and the gap in median achievement narrowed from 4.0% to 0.8% during this period. Increase in achievement during this time was inversely associated with practice performance in previous years (p < 0.0001) but was not associated with area deprivation (p = 0.062)
Millett (2007): Impact of a pay-for-performance incentive on support for smoking cessation and on smoking prevalence among people with diabetes.[109]	Diabetes	2003–05	Longitudinal cross-sectional survey	Wandsworth Prospective Diabetes Study	32 general practices in Wandsworth	The reduction in the prevalence of smoking over the study period was lower among women [adjusted odds ratio (OR): 0.71; 95% CI: 0.53–0.95] but was not significantly different in the most and least affluent groups. In 2005,

						smoking rates continued to differ significantly with age (10.6–25.1%), sex (women, 11.5%; men, 20.6%) and ethnic background (4.9–24.9%)
McGovern (2008): The effect of the UK incentive-based contract on the management of patients with coronary heart disease in primary care.[110]	CHD	2004–05	Serial cross-sectional study	SPICE	310 general practices in Scotland	Post-contract, disparities between patient subgroups continued for certain components of care. Women were less likely to be recorded than men in nine of 11 components of care, with older patients (seven of 11 components of care) and the most deprived (four of 11 components of care) also less likely to have a record than the youngest and least deprived, respectively
Simpson (2006): Effect of the UK incentive-based contract on the management of patients with stroke in primary care.[111]	Stroke or transient ischemic attack	2004–05	Serial cross-sectional study	SPICE	310 general practices in Scotland	There was a large increase in the documentation of quality indicators among the oldest patients (>75 years) and the most affluent patients. This tended to attenuate age groups differences and to exacerbate differences between

(Continued)

TABLE 4.4 Impact of the QOF on equity: description of studies reviewed (Continued)

First author and paper	Condition	Study time period	Design	Data source	Sample size and setting	Results
						deprivation groups. Women tended to have larger increases in documentation than men; however, sex differences persisted, with women less likely than men to have smoking habits recorded (adjusted OR: 0.87; 95% CI: 0.81–0.95) or to receive anti-platelet or anti-coagulant therapy (adjusted OR: 0.93; 95% CI: 0.86–0.99)
Ashworth (2008): Effect of social deprivation on blood pressure monitoring and control in England: a survey of data from the Quality and Outcomes Framework.[112]	Blood pressure	2005–07	Retrospective longitudinal survey	QOF data	8515 general practices in England	The initial gap of 1.7% between mean blood pressure recording levels in practices located in the least deprived fifth of communities compared with the most deprived fifth, narrowed to 0.2% 3 years later. Achievement of target blood pressure levels in 2005 for practices located in the least deprived communities ranged from 71.0% (95% CI: 70.4–71.6%) for diabetes to 85.1% (84.7% to 85.6%) for CHD; practices in the most deprived communities achieved 68.9% (68.4% to 69.5%)

Millett (2007): Ethnic disparities in diabetes management and pay-for-performance in the UK: The Wandsworth prospective diabetes study.[113]	Diabetes	2003–06	Retrospective longitudinal study	Wandsworth Prospective Diabetes Study data	32 general practices in Wandsworth	The increases in the reached targets for HbA1c, BP and total cholesterol were broadly uniform across ethnic groups, except for the black Caribbean group, which had improvements in HbA1c and BP control that were significantly lower than in the white British group. Variations in prescribing and achievement of treatment targets between ethnic groups evident in 2003 were not attenuated in 2005

and 81.8% (81.3–82.3%), respectively. Three years later, target achievement in the least deprived practices had risen to 78.6% (78.1–79.1%) and 89.4% (89.1–89.7%), respectively. Target achievement in the most deprived practices rose similarly, to 79.2% (78.8–79.6%) and 88.4% (88.2–88.7%), respectively. Similar changes were observed for the achievement of blood pressure targets in hypertension, cerebrovascular disease and chronic kidney disease

(Continued)

TABLE 4.4 Impact of the QOF on equity: description of studies reviewed (Continued)

First author and paper	Condition	Study time period	Design	Data source	Sample size and setting	Results
Millett (2009): Impact of pay-for-performance on ethnic disparities in intermediate outcomes for diabetes: a longitudinal study.[114]	Diabetes	2000–05	Retrospective longitudinal study	Wandsworth Prospective Diabetes Study data	15 general practices in Battersea and Wandsworth South	After the introduction of the P4P incentive, reductions in mean systolic and diastolic blood pressure were significantly greater than predicted by underlying trends in improvement. Reductions in A1C levels were significantly greater than those predicted by the underlying trend in the white group (−0.5%) but not in the black (−0.3%) or South Asian (−0.4%) groups. Ethnic group disparities in annual measurement of blood pressure and A1C were abolished before the introduction of P4P
Ashworth (2007): The relationship between social deprivation and the quality of primary care: a national survey using the indicators from the UK Quality and Outcomes Framework.[115]	Multiple conditions	2004–06	Serial cross-sectional study	QOF data	8480 (2004–05) and 8264 practices (2005–06) general practices in England	Overall differences between primary care quality in deprived and prosperous communities were small. Geographical differences were less in group and training practices

Millett (2008): Ethnic disparities in coronary heart disease management and pay-for-performance in the UK.[116]	CHD	2003–05	Serial cross-sectional survey	General practice records	32 general practices in Wandsworth	Improvements in blood pressure control were greater in the black group compared with whites, with disparities evident at baseline being attenuated (black 54.8% vs. white 58.3% reaching target in 2005). Lower recording of blood pressure in the south Asian group evident in 2003 was attenuated in 2005. Statin prescribing remained significantly lower ($p < 0.001$) in the black group compared with the south Asian and white groups after the implementation of P4P (black 74.8%, south Asian 83.8% and white 80.2% in 2005)
McGovern (2008): Introduction of a new incentive and target-based contract for family physicians in the UK: good for older patients with diabetes but less good for women?[117]	Diabetes	2004–05	Serial cross-sectional study	SPICE	310 general practices in Scotland	One year post-contract women were less likely than men to have HbA(1c) (OR: 0.85; 95% CI: 0.80–0.91), serum creatinine (OR: 0.90; 95% CI: 0.84–0.96) and cholesterol recorded (OR: 0.83; 95% CI: 0.77–0.90) or achieve HbA(1c) (≤10.0%; OR: 0.87; 95% CI: 0.82–0.91) and cholesterol targets (≤5.0 mmol/L; OR: 0.83; 95% CI: 0.77–0.90)

Achievement of non-incentivised quality indicators

A national survey of care in 2004 found that indicator achievement in QOF conditions was 75%, compared with 58% in non-QOF conditions.[63] A study comparing changes in care for incentivised and non-incentivised conditions from 2003 to 2005 found that baseline care for non-incentivised conditions was much lower (35%) than for incentivised conditions (75%) and did not change with the introduction of the contract.[64] This finding may reflect the fact that the non-incentivised conditions had received less policy attention before the QOF, and there may not have been an underlying improvement trend in these conditions. A study of prescribing data from Scotland also looked at non-QOF interventions and found that prescribing of QOF drugs increased significantly faster than non-QOF drugs both before and after the introduction of the new contract.[65]

Health outcomes

Most studies show little relationship between QOF achievement and health service activity or health outcomes (*see* Table 4.1). Associations between QOF scores for six conditions and emergency admissions and mortality were small and inconsistent[66]; no association was found between QOF CHD scores and CHD admissions in all primary care trusts in England[67]; and no associations were found between QOF stroke scores and adherence to stroke guidance from the Royal College of Physicians[68] or between QOF achievement and adherence to British Thoracic Society spirometry standards.[69] However, there was a significant positive relationship between QOF scores for epilepsy seizure-free patients and epilepsy-related emergency hospitalisation.[70]

A modelling study estimated that the potential reduction in mortality from full implementation of the contract might have been 416/100 000 people per year in 2004/05 and 451 in 2006/07. In 2004/05, the potential reduction in mortality per 100 000 people per year ranged from 163 in CHD to eight in asthma.[71] Importantly, these numbers did not take account of any pre-contract activity, and so the actual gain from the contract implementation would have been considerably less. An earlier model of the potential benefits of treating cardiovascular disease in the QOF allowed for baseline treatment and estimated that 29 events per 10 000 people per 5 years could be prevented by reaching cholesterol-reduction targets (15 in CHD, seven in stroke and seven in diabetes).[72] An additional 15 events could be prevented by achieving blood pressure control targets in hypertensive patients.

Impact on professionals

There has been concern that an unintended consequence of the QOF might be to reduce the professionalism and 'internal motivation' of doctors, and so crowd out the caring aspect of consultations (*see* Table 4.2).[73,74] There is no evidence that the internal motivation of general practitioners has been damaged,[75] although doctors were more enthusiastic about targets that were aligned with professional priorities.[76,77] Both doctors and nurses have reported concerns about the emergence of a 'dual agenda' in consultations, with less time for holistic care, patients' concerns and non-incentivised care and a perceived loss of continuity of care.[78,79,80] They were also concerned about increasing use of templates or 'box-ticking' to manage performance.[81,82,83,84]

Cost consequences

A study comparing estimated mortality gain from eight preventive interventions with the estimated QOF payments for those interventions concluded that there was no relationship between pay and health gain (*see* Table 4.3).[89] A larger study by the University of York identified cost effectiveness evidence for 12 indicators in the 2006 revised contract with direct therapeutic effect.[90] The three most cost-effective indicators were using angiotensin-converting enzyme inhibitors or angiotensin receptor blockers for chronic kidney disease, anti-coagulant therapy for atrial fibrillation and beta-blockers for CHD. The per-patient payment in 2004/05 ranged from £0.13 (for a chronic kidney disease indicator) to £87.79 (for a mental health indicator). The cost effectiveness of an indicator varied by its baseline achievement, with generally smaller changes needed for an indicator to be cost-effective at low baseline uptake than at higher baselines. The authors urged caution in interpreting their results for a number of reasons, particularly the major uncertainties in the cost and QALY evidence and uncertainty about the generalisability of estimates to the United Kingdom.

Impact on equity

Health inequalities are a major policy and public health concern.[93] Six papers describing studies with a longitudinal or serial cross-sectional design with points of measurement before and after April 2004 were identified (*see* Table 4.4).[94,95,96,97,98,99] Four additional papers describing serial cross-sectional studies were included.[100,101,102,103] Before the introduction of the QOF, the evidence about inequalities in healthcare was mixed. Achievement of some indicators was lower for some groups, e.g., for older patients with CHD,[104] and for female and older patients with a recording or stroke or TIA.[105] However, there were no significant differences in care in other areas, e.g., smoking cessation advice rates in deprived and affluent groups,[106] and sometimes better care was recorded for minority groups, such as better monitoring of blood pressure in black patients.[107]

As discussed earlier, quality of care generally improved over time around the introduction of the QOF, and while all groups benefited from this improvement, the relative rate of improvement differed between groups. The resulting changes in inequalities over time are small, variable and dependent on the indicator, the level of achievement before the QOF, and the demographic variable (age, sex, socioeconomic status and ethnicity). However, some general patterns can be identified.

First, the gaps in care between different age groups for CHD, diabetes and cerebrovascular disease (CVD) were attenuated after QOF due to greater improvement in the worse off. For quality indicators with lower achievement for older than younger people, in the three studies from Scotland, there were greater improvements for older people in some but not all indicators.[118,119,120] For the minority of indicators in which achievement was higher in older people than younger before the QOF, the advantage either persisted[121,122] or disappeared because of the levelling up of the care for younger groups.[123]

Second, the gaps between achievement scores for men and women persisted or sometimes increased. Before the introduction of the contract, the studies from Scotland report that achievement scores were significantly higher for men than women for two of eight diabetes indicators, seven of 11 CHD indicators and seven of nine CVD indicators.[124,125,126] After the QOF, higher achievement for men was found again for nearly all these indicators and for an additional two of 11 CHD and three of eight diabetes indicators.[127,123,129] However, care improved more for women than men in one CHD indicator[130] and for the recording of the smoking status of patients with diabetes.[131]

Third, the gaps in achievement between the most and least deprived areas have been attenuated in England. The results differ between the studies of 310 practices in Scotland, and those using national data in England. In England, the existing gap in the first year after the introduction of the QOF narrowed and almost disappeared in the years after.[132,133,134] Interestingly, improvements in achievement were associated with worse practice performance previously, and not with area deprivation.[135] Nevertheless, in individual indicators large differences remain (e.g., for five of the 147 measured QOF quality indicators, the difference between the least and most deprived areas is larger than 10%[136]), and the poorest performing practices remain concentrated in the most deprived areas.[137]

Results from a smaller dataset of 310 practices in Scotland show a slightly different picture. Before the QOF, lower achievement was found in more deprived areas for a relatively small number of quality indicators related to CHD, diabetes and CVD (e.g., one of 11 indicators for CHD), and for some indicators achievement was higher in more deprived areas (e.g., achieving cholesterol target).[138,139,140] After the introduction of the QOF achievement for some indicators improved less in the most deprived areas (e.g., an additional inequity for three of nine CVD indicators), leading to bigger inequality in care.[141]

Fourth, the impact of QOF implementation differs by ethnic group. Both before and after the implementation of the QOF, the results regarding ethnic differences are variable. Studies focus mainly on CHD and diabetes. Before the QOF, South Asian patients with CHD had better controlled cholesterol than white or black patients, and afterwards they scored better in three additional aspects of care. The gaps in CHD achievement between black and white people reduced after implementation of the QOF in some but not all indicators.[142] Pre-QOF variations in achievement of diabetes indicators between ethnic groups were not attenuated in 2005.[143]

CONCLUSIONS
Summary of impact of the QOF

The reported achievement of QOF indicators was high in the first year of the contract and has risen further each year since. These improvements have taken place against a background trend of improving quality of primary care for many conditions in the QOF. Beyond that, it is difficult to draw firm conclusions about the effects of the QOF, despite the increasing number of publications. There have been no evaluations of the QOF using an experimental design, and the observational approach used in all the studies reported here limits any conclusions that can be drawn about whether the QOF caused any observed associated changes in outcomes. The diverse nature of the research means that it is not possible to synthesise data from different studies to produce an overall aggregated result about the impact of the QOF.

Bearing these caveats in mind, two tentative conclusions can be drawn from this review, albeit in need of confirmation from further research. First, performance after the QOF has been roughly in line with the trend predicted from the years before the QOF. Second, at least some QOF interventions have probably been cost-effective and equity enhancing. However, there is considerable variability at individual indicator level. Professionals feel consultations and continuity of care have suffered to some extent. There is very little research about patients' views of the impact of the QOF, or about the aspects of general practice not measured in the QOF, such as caring, context and the management of complexity and multiple conditions.

The achievements reported from national QOF data have also been reported from other sources, especially for diabetes, and so it is likely that there have been real gains in quality, rather than simply better recording of existing care.[144,145] The evidence about improvements relative to underlying trends is mixed, with some evidence for performance slightly above predicted trend (e.g., meeting blood pressure targets), and some evidence for performance slightly below trend. The mixed results should be expected given the range of conditions studied in different practices, and the uncertainties around modelling trends. It is not known whether pre-2004 upward trends would have continued in the absence of the QOF or tailed off, and if they continued, whether they would have remained linear as they approached the ceiling of 100% achievement.

The conditions incentivised in the first year of the QOF are different from other non-incentivised conditions in at least two ways. First, they have been well-researched and are relatively straightforward to measure. Second, they have been subject to previous national policy interventions such as National Service Frameworks[146] and NICE guidelines,[147] and so were generally well-managed before the QOF. There is no evidence that non-incentivised conditions were neglected any more after the QOF than they were before.

It is not surprising that almost no links have been found between QOF scores and hospital admissions and mortality, given the wide range of other factors associated with these outcomes, and the variable timescales. The exception is epilepsy, where the link between the QOF indicator (epilepsy seizure-free patients) and the related outcome (epilepsy-related emergency hospitalisation) has been found to be good.

The qualitative studies of professionals broadly agree that dealing with the QOF has taken some attention away from dealing with patients' concerns, and continuity of care may have suffered.

And what about cost? The QOF has been very expensive, and the single study of cost effectiveness cautiously offers some reassurance that it may have been worthwhile, at least for the 12 indicators studied with direct therapeutic effect. This has some support from evidence that a diabetes P4P programme delivered a return on investment, albeit in a very different context in the United States.[148]

The lack of equity-related theoretical and conceptual rigour in the studies and important methodological limitations such as the lack of data on the non-users of the healthcare system, make assessing the equity dimension of the QOF very difficult. There are a number of possible explanations for the more consistent picture of reducing inequalities by area deprivation seen in the national English data than in the Scottish studies. The results may be sensitive to the measure of quality used,[149] or the subset of practices studied may be different from other practices nationally. In England, the findings from local and national studies are inconsistent, with local studies of QOF indicators and deprivation reporting either no association between quality and deprivation, or better quality in more deprived areas.[150,151,152,153]

Further research

Good quality healthcare should be effective, efficient, safe, timely, equitable and patient centred.[154] As noted earlier, the biggest gap in the research reviewed here is in patients' and users' views of the QOF. There is also a need for more research into the non-incentivised aspects of the QOF, which in turn requires the development of better measures for those important aspects of care that are currently unmeasurable or unmeasured. Studies are needed that address implementation of the QOF from a broader theoretical perspective of equity, including distinguishing between horizontal (i.e., equitable care for individual patients) and vertical (i.e., equitable care for conditions) equity, and between equal access, treatment and outcomes for equal need.[155] There is a need for databases linking individual data over the years, rather than serial cross-sectional studies and for individual rather than area-based measures of socio-economic status.

There is uncertainty about the organisation of the QOF: how big should the financial rewards be? How low or high should achievement thresholds be set for payment, given that baseline achievement for many indicators was already above thresholds for maximum payment,[156] and that non-eligible patients can be excepted from indicators?[157] What proportion of the total incentive payment should be attached to patient measures of quality, rather than self-reported data?[158] How should conditions be chosen for inclusion in the QOF, and for retirement from the QOF? What will happen to performance after an indicator is retired? Should the size of reward be determined by potential population health gain or by the work-load for primary care professionals?

Implications

Evaluating the impact of a major policy initiative such as the QOF is important in order to inform future health policy development. The tentative conclusions of this require further research to strengthen or refute them, but as important is a forward-looking research agenda. The QOF is likely to be with us for some time to come. NICE will have to decide on developments to the clinical and health improvement indicators for the QOF[159] – whether or not evidence is available. This review has sug-gested some areas where future research efforts could usefully be targeted.

REFERENCES

1. Steel N, Bachmann M, Maisey S, *et al.* Self reported receipt of care consistent with 32 quality indicators: national population survey of adults aged 50 or more in England. *BMJ.* 2008; **337**: a957.
2. McGlynn EA, Asch SM, Adams J, *et al.* The quality of health care delivered to adults in the United States. *N Engl J Med.* 2003; **348**(26): 2635–45.
3. General Practitioners Committee BMA, The NHS Confederation. *Investing in General Practice: the new General Medical Services contract.* London: The NHS Confederation; 2003.
4. NHS Employers and the General Practitioners Committee. *Quality and Outcomes Framework guidance for GMS contract 2009/10: delivering investment in general practice.* London: NHS Employers; 2009.
5. Ibid.
6. Roland M. Linking physicians' pay to the quality of care—a major experiment in the United Kingdom. *N Engl J Med.* 2004; **351**(14): 1448–54.
7. Annemans L, Boeckxstaens P, Borgermans L, *et al.* Voordelen, nadelen en haalbaar-heid van het invoeren van 'Pay for Quality' programma's in België [Advantages, dis-advantages and feasibility of the introduction of 'Pay for Quality' programmes in Belgium]. KCE report 118A. Suppl. 118S ed. Brussel: Federaal Kenniscentrum voor de Gezondheidszorg [Belgian Health Care Knowledge Centre]; 2009.
8. Christianson J, Leatherman S, Sutherland K. *Financial Incentives, Healthcare Providers and Quality Improvements: a review of the evidence.* London: The Health Foundation; 2007.
9. National Institute for Health and Clinical Excellence. *About the Quality and Outcomes Framework (QOF);* 2010 [cited 20 Jan 2010]. Available at: www.nice.org.uk/about-nice/qof/qof.jsp

10. Donabedian A. Explorations in quality assessment and monitoring. In: Donabedian A, editor. *The Definition of Quality and Approaches to its Assessment.* Vol. 1. Ann Arbor, MI: Health Administration Press; 1980.

11. Annemans, Boeckxstaens, Borgermans, *et al.,* op. cit.

12. Christianson, Leatherman, Sutherland, op. cit.

13. Roland M. *Comment on 'Financial Incentives, Healthcare Providers and Quality Improvements'.* London: The Health Foundation; 2010.

14. Doran T, Fullwood C, Gravelle H, *et al.* Pay-for-performance programs in family practices in the United Kingdom. *N Engl J Med.* 2006; **355**(4): 375–84.

15. Doran T, Fullwood C, Reeves D, *et al.* Exclusion of patients from pay-for-performance targets by English physicians. *New Engl J Med.* 2008; **359**(3): 274–84.

16. Doran T, Fullwood C, Kontopantelis E, *et al.* Effect of financial incentives on inequalities in the delivery of primary clinical care in England: analysis of clinical activity indicators for the Quality and Outcomes Framework. *Lancet.* 2008; **372**(9640): 728–36.

17. Fleetcroft R, Parekh S, Steel N, *et al.* Potential population health gain of the Quality and Outcomes Framework. In: *Quality and Outcomes Framework. Joint executive summary: Reports to the Department of Health.* University of East Anglia and University of York; 2008.

18. MacBride-Stewart SP, Elton R, *et al.* Do quality incentives change prescribing patterns in primary care? An observational study in Scotland. *Fam Pract.* 2008; **25**(1): 27–32.

19. Downing A, Rudge G, Cheng Y, *et al.* Do the UK government's new Quality and Outcomes Framework (QOF) scores adequately measure primary care performance? A cross-sectional survey of routine healthcare data. *BMC Health Serv Res.* 2007; **7**(1): 166.

20. Hippisley-Cox J, Vinogradova Y, Coupland C. *Final Report for the Information Centre for Health and Social Care: time series analysis for 2001–2006 for selected clinical indicators from the Quality and Outcomes Framework;* 2007.

21. Campbell S, Reeves D, Kontopantelis E, *et al.* Quality of primary care in England with the introduction of pay for performance. *New Engl J Med.* 2007; **357**(2): 181–90.

22. Steel N, Maisey S, Clark A, *et al.* Quality of clinical primary care and targeted incentive payments: an observational study. *Br J Gen Pract.* 2007; **57**: 449–54.

23. Gulliford MC, Ashworth M, Robotham D, *et al.* Achievement of metabolic targets for diabetes by English primary care practices under a new system of incentives. *Diabet Med.* 2007; **24**(5): 505–11.

24. Khunti K, Gadsby R, Millett C, *et al.* Quality of diabetes care in the UK: comparison of published quality-of-care reports with results of the Quality and Outcomes Framework for diabetes. *Diabet Med.* 2007; **24**(12): 1436–41.

25. Calvert M, Shankar A, McManus RJ, *et al.* Effect of the Quality and Outcomes Framework on diabetes care in the United Kingdom: retrospective cohort study. *BMJ.* 2009; **338**(2): b1870.

26. Srirangalingam U, Sahathevan SK, Lasker SS, *et al.* Changing pattern of referral to a diabetes clinic following implementation of the new UK GP Contract. *Br J Gen Pract.* 2006; **56**(529): 624–6.

27. Millett C, Gray J, Saxena S, *et al.* Impact of a pay-for-performance incentive on support for smoking cessation and on smoking prevalence among people with diabetes. *Can Med Assoc J.* 2007; **176**(12): 1705–10.

28. Jaiveer PK, Jaiveer S, Jujjavarapu SB, *et al.* Improvements in clinical diabetes care in the first year of the new General Medical Services contract in the UK. *Br J Diab Vasc Dis.* 2006; **6**(1): 45–8.

29. McGovern M, Williams D, Hannaford P, *et al.* Introduction of a new incentive and target-based contract for family physicians in the UK: good for older patients with diabetes but less good for women? *Diabet Med.* 2008; **25**(9): 1083–9.

30. Millett C, Bottle A, Ng A, *et al.* Pay for performance and the quality of diabetes management in individuals with and without co-morbid medical conditions. *J R Soc Med.* 2009; **102**(9): 369–77.

31. Tahrani AA, McCarthy M, Godson J, *et al.* Diabetes care and the new GMS contract: the evidence for a whole county. *Br J Gen Pract.* 2007; **57**(539): 483–5.

32. Tahrani AA, McCarthy M, Godson J, *et al.* Impact of practice size on delivery of diabetes care before and after the Quality and Outcomes Framework implementation. *Br J Gen Pract.* 2008; **58**(553): 576–9.

33. Vaghela P, Ashworth M, Schofield P, *et al.* Population intermediate outcomes of diabetes under pay-for-performance incentives in England from 2004 to 2008. *Diabetes Care.* 2009; **32**(3): 427–9.

34. Bottle A, Gnani S, Saxena S, *et al.* Association between quality of primary care and hospitalization for coronary heart disease in England: national cross-sectional study. *J Gen Intern Med.* 2008; **23**(2): 135–41.

35. McGovern MP, Boroujerdi MA, Taylor MW, *et al.* The effect of the UK incentive-based contract on the management of patients with coronary heart disease in primary care. *Fam Pract.* 2008; **25**(1): 33–9.

36. Williams PH, de Lusignan S. Does a higher 'quality points' score mean better care in stroke? An audit of general practice medical records. *Inform Prim Care.* 2006; **14**(1): 29–40.

37. Simpson CR, Hannaford PC, Lefevre K, *et al.* Effect of the UK incentive-based contract on the management of patients with stroke in primary care. *Stroke.* 2006; **37**(9): 2354–60.

38. McElduff P, Lyratzopoulos G, Edwards R, *et al.* Will changes in primary care improve health outcomes? Modelling the impact of financial incentives introduced to improve quality of care in the UK. *Qual Saf Health Care.* 2004; **13**(3): 191–7.

39. Ashworth M, Medina J, Morgan M. Effect of social deprivation on blood pressure monitoring and control in England: a survey of data from the Quality and Outcomes Framework. *BMJ.* 2008; **337**(2): a2030.

40. Shohet C, Yelloly J, Bingham P, *et al.* The association between the quality of epilepsy management in primary care, general practice population deprivation status and epilepsy-related emergency hospitalisations. *Seizure.* 2007; **16**(4): 351–5.

41. Coleman T, Lewis S, Hubbard R, *et al.* Impact of contractual financial incentives on the ascertainment and management of smoking in primary care. *Addiction.* 2007; **102**(5): 803–8.

42. Strong M, South G, Carlisle R. The UK Quality and Outcomes Framework pay-for-performance scheme and spirometry: rewarding quality or just quantity? A cross-sectional study in Rotherham, UK. *BMC Health Serv Res.* 2009; **9**(1): 108.

43. Doran T, Fullwood C, Gravelle H, *et al.*, op. cit.

44. Doran T, Fullwood C, Kontopantelis E, *et al.*, op. cit.

45. Doran T, Fullwood C, Reeves D, *et al.*, op. cit.

46. Vaghela P, Ashworth M, Schofield P, *et al.*, op. cit.
47. Khunti K, Gadsby R, Millett C, *et al.*, op. cit.
48. McGovern, Williams, Hannaford, *et al.*, op. cit.
49. Millett C, Gray J, Saxena S, *et al.*, op. cit.
50. Jaiveer, Jaiveer, Jujjavarapu, *et al.*, op. cit.
51. Tahrani, McCarthy, Godson, *et al.*, op. cit.
52. Tahrani, McCarthy, Godson, *et al.*, op. cit.
53. Srirangalingam, Sahathevan, Lasker, *et al.*, op. cit.
54. McGovern, Boroujerdi, Taylor, *et al.*, op. cit.
55. Simpson, Hannaford, Lefevre, *et al.*, op. cit.
56. Ashworth, Medina, Morgan, op. cit.
57. Coleman, Lewis, Hubbard, *et al.*, op. cit.
58. Hippisley-Cox, Vinogradova, Coupland, op. cit.
59. Campbell, Reeves, Kontopantelis, *et al.*, op. cit.
60. Gulliford, Ashworth, Robotham, *et al.*, op. cit.
61. Millett, Bottle, Ng, *et al.*, op. cit.
62. Calvert, Shankar, McManus, *et al.*, op. cit.
63. Steel, Bachmann, Maisey, *et al.*, op. cit.
64. Steel, Maisey, Clark, *et al.*, op. cit.
65. MacBride-Stewart, Elton, Walley, op. cit.
66. Downing, Rudge, Cheng, op. cit.
67. Bottle, Gnani, Saxena, *et al.*, op. cit.
68. Williams, de Lusignan, op. cit.
69. Strong, South, Carlisle, op. cit.
70. Shohet, Yelloly, Bingham, *et al.*, op. cit.
71. Fleetcroft, Parekh, Steel, *et al.*, op. cit.
72. McElduff, Lyratzopoulos, Edwards, *et al.*, op. cit.
73. Mangin D, Toop L. The Quality and Outcomes Framework: what have you done to yourselves? *Br J Gen Pract.* 2007; **57**(539): 435–7.
74. Marshall M, Harrison S. It's about more than money: financial incentives and internal motivation. *Qual Saf Health Care.* 2005; **14**(1): 4–5.
75. McDonald R, Harrison S, Checkland K, *et al.* Impact of financial incentives on clinical autonomy and internal motivation in primary care: ethnographic study. *BMJ.* 2007; **334**(7608): 1357.
76. Campbell SM, McDonald R, Lester H. The experience of pay for performance in English family practice: a qualitative study. *Ann Fam Med.* 2008; **6**(3): 228–34.
77. Maisey S, Steel N, Marsh R, *et al.* Effects of payment for performance in primary care: qualitative interview study. *J Health Serv Res Policy.* 2008; **13**(3): 133–9.
78. Campbell, McDonald, Lester, op. cit.
79. Maisey, Steel, Marsh, *et al.*, op. cit.
80. McGregor W, Jabareen H, O'Donnell CA, *et al.* Impact of the 2004 GMS contract on practice nurses: a qualitative study. *Br J Gen Pract.* 2008; **58**(555): 711–19.
81. McDonald, Harrison, Checkland, *et al.*, op. cit.
82. Campbell, McDonald, Lester, op. cit.
83. Maisey, Steel, Marsh, *et al.*, op. cit.
84. McGregor, Jabareen, O'Donnell, *et al.*, op. cit.
85. Campbell, McDonald, Lester, op. cit.
86. Maisey, Steel, Marsh, *et al.*, op. cit.

87. McDonald, Harrison, Checkland, *et al.*, op. cit.

88. McGregor, Jabareen, O'Donnell, *et al.*, op. cit.

89. Fleetcroft R, Cookson R. Do the incentive payments in the new NHS contract for primary care reflect likely population health gains? *J Health Serv Res Policy.* 2006; **11**(1): 27–31.

90. Mason A, Walker S, Claxton K, *et al.* The GMS Quality and Outcomes Framework: are the Quality and Outcomes Framework (QOF) indicators a cost-effective use of NHS resources? In: *Quality and Outcomes Framework. Joint executive summary: Reports to the Department of Health.* University of East Anglia and University of York; 2008.

91. Mason, Walker, Claxton, *et al.*, op. cit.

92. Fleetcroft, Cookson, op. cit.

93. The Marmot Review. *Fair Society, Healthy Lives. Strategic Review of Health Inequalities in England post-2010.* London: The Marmot Review; 2010.

94. Millett, Gray, Saxena, *et al.*, op. cit.

95. Ashworth, Medina, Morgan, op. cit.

96. Millett C, Gray J, Saxena S, *et al.* Ethnic disparities in diabetes management and pay-for-performance in the UK: The Wandsworth prospective diabetes study. *PLoS Med.* 2007; **4**(6): 1087–93.

97. Millett C, Netuveli G, Saxena S, *et al.* Impact of pay for performance on ethnic disparities in intermediate outcomes for diabetes: a longitudinal study. *Diabetes Care.* 2009; **32**(3): 404–9.

98. Ashworth M, Seed P, Armstrong D, *et al.* The relationship between social deprivation and the quality of primary care: a national survey using indicators from the UK Quality and Outcomes Framework. *Br J Gen Pract.* 2007; **57**(539): 441–8.

99. Millett C, Gray J, Wall M, *et al.* Ethnic disparities in coronary heart disease management and pay for performance in the UK. *J Gen Intern Med.* 2008; **24**(1): 8–13.

100. Doran, Fullwood, Kontopantelis, *et al.*, op. cit.

101. McGovern, Boroujerdi, Taylor, *et al.*, op. cit.

102. Simpson, Hannaford, Lefevre, *et al.*, op. cit.

103. McGovern, Williams, Hannaford, *et al.*, op. cit.

104. McGovern, Boroujerdi, Taylor, *et al.*, op. cit.

105. Simpson, Hannaford, Lefevre, *et al.*, op. cit.

106. Millett, Gray, Saxena, *et al.*, op. cit.

107. Millett, Netuveli, Saxena, *et al.*, op. cit.

108. Doran, Fullwood, Kontopantelis, *et al.*, op. cit.

109. Millett, Gray, Saxena, *et al.*, op. cit.

110. McGovern, Boroujerdi, Taylor, *et al.*, op. cit.

111. Simpson, Hannaford, Lefevre, *et al.*, op. cit.

112. Ashworth, Medina, Morgan, op. cit.

113. Millett, Gray, Saxena, *et al.*, op. cit.

114. Millett, Netuveli, Saxena, *et al.*, op. cit.

115. Ashworth, Seed, Armstrong, *et al.*, op. cit.

116. Millett, Gray, Wall, *et al.*, op. cit.

117. McGovern, Williams, Hannaford, *et al.*, op. cit.

118. Ibid.

119. McGovern, Boroujerdi, Taylor, *et al.*, op. cit.

120. Simpson, Hannaford, Lefevre, *et al.*, op. cit.

121. McGovern, Williams, Hannaford, *et al.*, op. cit.
122. McGovern, Boroujerdi, Taylor, *et al.*, op. cit.
123. Millett, Gray, Saxena, *et al.*, op. cit.
124. McGovern, Williams, Hannaford, *et al.*, op. cit.
125. McGovern, Boroujerdi, Taylor, *et al.*, op. cit.
126. Simpson, Hannaford, Lefevre, *et al.*, op. cit.
127. McGovern, Williams, Hannaford, *et al.*, op. cit.
128. McGovern, Boroujerdi, Taylor, *et al.*, op. cit.
129. Simpson, Hannaford, Lefevre, *et al.*, op. cit.
130. McGovern, Boroujerdi, Taylor, *et al.*, op. cit.
131. Millett, Gray, Saxena, *et al.*, op. cit.
132. Doran, Fullwood, Kontopantelis, *et al.*, op. cit.
133. Ashworth, Medina, Morgan, op. cit.
134. Ashworth, Seed, Armstrong, *et al.*, op. cit.
135. Doran, Fullwood, Kontopantelis, *et al.*, op. cit.
136. Ashworth, Seed, Armstrong, *et al.*, op. cit.
137. Doran, Fullwood, Kontopantelis, *et al.*, op. cit.
138. McGovern, Williams, Hannaford, *et al.*, op. cit.
139. McGovern, Boroujerdi, Taylor, *et al.*, op. cit.
140. Simpson, Hannaford, Lefevre, *et al.*, op. cit.
141. Ibid.
142. Millett, Gray, Wall, *et al.*, op. cit.
143. Millett, Gray, Saxena, *et al.*, op. cit.
144. Steel, Bachmann, Maisey, *et al.*, op. cit.
145. Hippisley-Cox, Vinogradova, Coupland, op. cit.
146. Secretary of State for Health. *National Service Framework for Coronary Heart Disease. Modern Standards and Service Models.* London: Department of Health; 2000.
147. National Institute for Health and Clinical Excellence; 2010 [cited 28 Jan 2010]; Available at: www.nice.org.uk/
148. Curtin K, Beckman H, Pankow G, *et al.* Return on investment in pay for performance: a diabetes case study. *J Health Manag.* 2006; **51**(6): 365–74.
149. McLean G, Sutton M, Guthrie B. Deprivation and quality of primary care services: evidence for persistence of the inverse care law from the UK Quality and Outcomes Framework. *J Epidemiol Community Health.* 2006; **60**(11): 917–22.
150. Strong M, Maheswaran R, Radford J. Socioeconomic deprivation, coronary heart disease prevalence and quality of care: a practice-level analysis in Rotherham using data from the new UK general practitioner Quality and Outcomes Framework. *J Public Health.* 2006; **28**(1): 39–42.
151. Abdelhamid AS, Maisey S, Steel N. Predictors of the quality of care for asthma in general practice: an observational study. *Fam Pract.* 2010; **27**(2): 186–91.
152. Broadbent J, Maisey S, Holland R, *et al.* Recorded quality of primary care for osteoarthritis: an observational study. *Br J Gen Pract.* 2008; **58**(557): 839–43.
153. Vedavanam S, Steel N, Broadbent J, *et al.* Recorded quality of care for depression in general practice: an observational study. *Br J Gen Pract.* 2009; **59**: 94–8.
154. Institute of Medicine (IOM), Committee on Health Care in America. *Crossing the Quality Chasm: a new health system for the 21st century.* Washington, DC: National Academy Press; 2001.

155. Goddard M, Smith P. Equity of access to health care services: theory and evidence from the UK. *Soc Sci Med.* 2001; **53**(9): 1149–62.
156. Calvert, Shankar, McManus, *et al.*, op. cit.
157. Fleetcroft R, Steel N, Cookson R, *et al.* Mind the gap! Evaluation of the performance gap attributable to exception reporting and target thresholds in the new GMS contract: national database analysis. *BMC Health Serv Res.* 2008; **8**: 131.
158. Galvin R. Pay-for-performance: too much of a good thing? A conversation with Martin Roland. *Health Aff.* 2006; **25**(5): w412–9.
159. National Institute for Health and Clinical Excellence. *About the Quality and Outcomes Framework (QOF),* op. cit.

CHAPTER 5

The public health impact

Anna Dixon, Artak Khachatryan and Tammy Boyce

SUMMARY

Clear policy objectives encourage primary care and general practice to address health inequalities. In this chapter, we explore the potential impact of the Quality and Outcomes Framework (QOF) on health inequalities in more detail and review the available evidence including analysis of the area-based differences in performance between practices in Spearhead and non-Spearhead areas.

Overall, the evidence suggests that differences in performance, as measured by the QOF, between practices in deprived and non-deprived areas are narrowing. QOF achievement has improved in all practices. However, there is weak evidence as to the impact of the QOF on health. The evidence is equivocal as to whether improvements in clinical care and the narrowing gap in performance have been influenced by the incentives created by the QOF and whether this translates into reduced health inequalities.

Although the QOF is only one incentive that practices face, it is vital that indicators are aligned to the objective of reducing health inequalities. Additional research is needed to establish whether the QOF ensures that the 'hard to reach' and those with greater care needs are gaining access to high-quality primary care.

Key points
- Research demonstrates that there are small absolute differences between practices in performance on the QOF. Differences between the least and most deprived practices are gradually narrowing.
- There is limited evidence of the direct impact of the QOF on health or health inequalities. Improvements in some clinical areas predated the QOF.
- Our research suggests that the QOF may be having a small, positive impact on reducing area-based health inequalities, but area-based initiatives to tackle inequalities have not yet had an observable impact on deprived practices.

- The selection and weighting of the QOF indicators in future should be better aligned to the objective of reducing health inequalities.

INTRODUCTION

General practice and primary care, more broadly, has traditionally played a major role in public health. The model of general practice in the United Kingdom, whereby practices provide both primary and secondary prevention to an enrolled population supports this approach. Particularly in more deprived communities, primary care has often played a key role in promoting health and tackling the wider social determinants of health in an effort to reduce health inequalities.[1]

Several indicators in the Quality and Outcomes Framework (QOF) focus on clinical activities that contribute to public health. Although reducing health inequalities was not an explicit policy objective of the QOF, there has been growing interest in the impact of the QOF on public health and, specifically, on health inequalities.[2] In this chapter, we seek to examine the likely impact of the QOF on public health and health inequalities, reviewing the evidence from published work as well as drawing on our own research.

BACKGROUND

In 2001, the labour government set a series of ambitious targets to reduce health inequalities in England by 2010. These included targets to close the gap in life expectancy at birth, infant mortality and mortality from the major killers. Significant progress has been made in improving life expectancy in absolute terms across all social groups. The target to reduce by at least 10% the gap in life expectancy between the fifth of areas with the worst health and deprivation indicators (so-called Spearhead areas) and the population as a whole will not be met.[3] There are 62 primary care trusts (PCTs) in England, which are designated Spearhead PCTs [reduced from 88 following National Health Service (NHS) reconfiguration in 2006], for which addressing the causes of premature mortality has been a priority. Despite significant improvements in life expectancy in Spearhead PCTs, progress has been slower than in non-Spearhead areas. Consequently, the gap in life expectancy is actually widening. For males, the absolute gap in life expectancy between England and the group of Spearhead PCTs in 2006–08 was 2.1 years (compared with 1.9 in 1995–97, the baseline years for the purposes of the target) and for females 1.7 years compared with 1.4 years at baseline.[4] Thirty-seven of the 70 Spearhead local authority areas are 'off track' to narrow the relative gap in life expectancy with the England average by 10%.

Figure 5.1 shows the relative gap between England and the Spearhead average, which is the basis of the life expectancy national target.[5] The national target aimed at a 10% minimum reduction in relative gap, from 2.57% in 1995–97 (baseline) to 2.32% in 2009–11 for males, and from 1.77% in 1995–97 to 1.59% in 2009–11 for

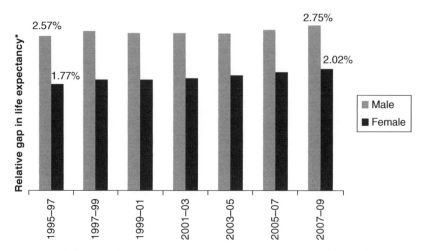

FIGURE 5.1 Relative gap in life expectancy between England and Spearhead group for males and females. *Differences in rates between England and Spearhead group as a percentage of the England rate

females. However, as the latest figures show, the relative gap between England and the Spearhead group was wider in 2007–09 than at baseline (1995–97), both for males (2.75% vs. 2.57%) and females (2.02% vs. 1.77%).[6]

As for the infant mortality target, the latest figures (2009) show that the gap between the population as a whole and the routine and manual groups has not reduced from the previous year and remains at 16%.[7] Therefore, achieving the national target of a 10% minimum reduction in relative gap, from 13% in 1997–99 (baseline) to 12% in 2009–11, is not likely to be met.

Although the overall targets are unlikely to be met, there has been varied success in meeting the targets across England. In many cases, non-Spearhead PCTs appear to be improving at a faster rate than Spearheads. For instance, in 2007/08 fewer Spearheads met the 4-week smoking quitters indicator than in 2006/07 while the number of non-Spearheads meeting this indicator improved.[8]

The Department of Health has recognised the important contribution of health-care and the NHS to tackling health inequalities. The health inequalities intervention tool (HIIT) was launched in 2007 to help Spearhead areas identify key drivers of health inequalities and interventions that would help PCTs to meet the targets. The HIIT focused heavily on the impact of smoking cessation, antihypertensive and statin prescribing. More recently, the Department of Health has estimated that car-diovascular disease [mainly coronary heart disease (CHD)], cancer and respiratory disease account for two-thirds of the gap and that the main interventions that can contribute to a reduction in the gap include: smoking cessation, control of blood pressure, cholesterol and high blood sugar in diabetics and anticoagulant therapy in patients with atrial fibrillation.[9] The strategies identified by the National Support Team for Health Inequalities also suggest an important role for primary care in reducing health inequalities. These include a proactive approach to identifying unmet need in primary care and ensuring the quality and quantity of primary care in disadvantaged areas are sufficient to meet local needs.[10]

The government has sought to reduce inequalities by tackling the wider determinants, initially through a cross-departmental programme of activities.[11] In 2008, the government established a strategic review of health inequalities led by Sir Michael Marmot to consider the approach needed to tackle health inequalities post-2010. The final recommendations of this report addressed the causes of health inequalities, emphasising the importance of good early years' support and education, the importance of education across all ages, good employment and a minimum income for healthy living.[12]

The report concluded, as did the Acheson report published in 1998, that there is a limit to what the NHS can achieve on its own and, as such, the majority of the Marmot Review's recommendations were targeted at stakeholders beyond the NHS and Department of Health. The report recommended that the NHS and Department of Health work in partnership with local authorities, schools and employers as well as other government departments to tackle the causes of health inequalities.

These policy objectives recommend that primary care and general practice can make a significant contribution to the reduction in health inequalities. Although reducing health inequalities was not one of its original aims, the Department of Health now regards it as one of the QOF's explicit goals.

THE POTENTIAL IMPACT OF THE QOF ON INEQUALITIES

Although the QOF was not explicitly designed to tackle health inequalities, its aim of improving general practitioner (GP) performance and reducing variations in the management of common chronic conditions has the potential to do so. However, as the Marmot review rightly indicated,[13] the introduction of the QOF also has the potential to increase health inequalities by diverting attention from non-incentivised conditions (*see* Box 5.1).

A number of assumptions need to hold true if general practice and, specifically the QOF, is to have a beneficial impact on reducing health inequalities. First, the QOF indicators must provide incentives for GPs and practices to undertake activities, which have a direct impact on an individual's health. Second, practices must be equally able to respond to the incentives and not face differential barriers in their ability to monitor and report activities (e.g., practices in poorer areas may have less investment in facilities, information technology or practice staff). Third, these activities must be more prevalent and/or increase more quickly in practices, which serve deprived populations or (for the purposes of the target) practices in Spearhead areas (regardless of the particular characteristics of the practice population). Fourth, these activities (which are targeted with incentives) must not crowd out other activities, which are more beneficial to population health. Fifth, practices must have

---

Box 5.1 Key points from the task group recommendations for the Marmot review on health inequalities[14]

- NICE reviews of both existing and potential new QOF indicators should include a formal and comprehensive assessment of their impact on health inequalities.
- More primary prevention-related indicators should be introduced in the QOF. (The QOF is only a part of more complex primary prevention activities within general practice.)
- The provision to 'exception report' patients should be retained.
- Annual reviews of maximum payment thresholds for the QOF corresponding to the patterns of achievement should be conducted.
- Possibility of 'retirement' of highly achieved indicators but with continuous follow-up should be considered.
- Data on non-QOF conditions should be routinely monitored.

---

incentives to case find, particularly in areas of known high disease prevalence, and to minimise the number of exceptional cases reported.

RESEARCH EVIDENCE
Socio-economic inequalities

Early analysis of the QOF found that differences in performance between general practices was small and declining.[15] A number of studies have specifically looked at the extent to which variation in performance differs significantly by deprivation.

Ashworth *et al.* analysed the first 2 years of QOF data, comparing mean total QOF scores between practices in the least and the most deprived quintiles.[16] Small differences were observed – 64.5 points difference in 2004/05; and 30.4 points difference in 2005/06. Doran *et al.* reported differences in QOF performance on a range of clinical indicators between the least and the most deprived practices but noted the gap had reduced from 4% to 0.88% between 2004/05 and 2006/07 years.[17] Other studies looking at specific indicators and conditions measured within the QOF have shown similar results, that is a narrowing in the gap between the least and the most deprived areas.[18]

Research has also sought to examine the extent to which deprivation explains variation in QOF achievement. Overall, there appears to be a weak negative correlation between QOF achievement and deprivation, most deprived practices are associated with lower achievement in the QOF. The strength and statistical significance of associations varies depending on the indicators assessed and practice factors considered, such as list size and caseload.

In a descriptive study of general practices within one English PCT, a weak negative (not statistically significant) correlation was found between overall QOF scores and deprivation scores.[19] Wang found that size of practice influenced the association between deprivation and performance, with smaller practices performing less well in relation to organisational indicators but performing as well for clinical ones.[20] Ashworth and Armstrong examined the relationship between QOF achievement, social deprivation and practice characteristics, using the first year of QOF data for England.[21] In a regression model, type of practices (i.e., whether they were training practices or group practices) and social deprivation explained around only 14.6% of the variation in QOF scores. Another study of general practices in England suggested that area deprivation may not be as important a factor as the practice performance in the previous year in predicting QOF achievement.[22]

National studies using data from England and Scotland examined the associations between quality in care for cardiovascular disease, as measured by QOF achievement, and general practice caseload, practice size and area-based deprivation.[23] They assessed practice achievement against 26 QOF indicators relating to cardiovascular disease including indicators in the clinical domains of CHD, left ventricular dysfunction and stroke. Statistically significant associations were found only for indicators requiring referral for further investigation ($p < 0.01$).

Evidence suggests that differences in exception reporting are not significantly associated with deprivation (statistical significance at $p < 0.05$)[24] and the differences between practice prevalence (as measured by disease registers within the QOF) and population prevalence (as measured by population surveys) appear to be narrowing. However, there remains some concern that the practices in deprived areas face a disincentive to actively case find than practices in affluent areas with lower prevalence.[25] In response to such concerns, the government has committed to ensure that QOF payments are fully adjusted to reflect relative disease prevalence.[26] Up until 2009, the QOF payment system discriminated against practices with high disease prevalence, frequently concentrated in deprived areas: they received less remuneration per patient than those with low prevalence.[27]

IMPACT ON HEALTH

As noted earlier, the QOF includes a range of indicators only some of which are clinical and therefore are likely to have a direct impact on health. Fleetcroft and Cookson identified a subset of indicators that measure practice achievement on aspects of activity, which could potentially contribute to health gain (38 out of a total of 81 clinical indicators).[28] Further work to inform the selection of new QOF indicators undertaken by researchers at York University and the University of East Anglia (UEA) has sought to calculate lives saved and the cost effectiveness of the QOF using evidence from published controlled trials for each of the clinical indicators.[29] They estimated that the potential lives saved per 100 000 population per year had increased from 415.77 (400.32–444.99) in the 2003 contract to 451.5

(423.98–480.72) in the 2006 contract across all clinical indicators and domains. The domains of CHD and diabetes had the most potential lives saved – 160.9 and 107.1 respectively – with other domains having potential to save less than 50 lives and smoking cessation just 10.9 lives per 100 000.[30]

Other studies have linked QOF data with clinical data in order to assess the impact on health. Studies that have linked QOF data with hospital admission figures suggest that while higher clinical QOF scores are generally associated with lower hospital admission rates, the strength and significance of associations varied geographically and by clinical condition assessed. Deprivation was shown to be more strongly correlated with admission rates than QOF scores.[31,32] Discrepancies between adherence to clinical guidelines and QOF achievement for particular conditions have also been observed.[33,34]

In general, as Kordowicz and Ashworth attest in Chapter 6, the evidence is equivocal on whether improvements in clinical care and the narrowing gap in performance are influenced by the incentives created by the QOF. Time series analysis of selected clinical indicators suggests that improvements may have predated the introduction of the QOF, although the rate of improvement has continued since that time.[35] A systematic review of the literature indicated a modest improvement in diabetes care since the introduction of the QOF.[36] The quality of chronic disease management (CHD, diabetes and hypertension – in terms of blood pressure and cholesterol targets) in England was broadly equitable between socio-economic groups before the QOF's introduction, and remained so after its introduction.[37] In a study of achievement of metabolic targets following introduction of the QOF, Gulliford *et al.* concluded that, while financial incentives may have contributed to the improvement of services and clinical outcomes, there remained a deprivation gap in achievement of targets (around 3% lower achievement in the most deprived areas).[38] For some conditions covered by the QOF, there is evidence of excessive or inappropriate prescriptions or referrals.[39,40,41] Although quality of care for some non-incentivised activities was improving before 2004, it does not appear to have continued to improve after introduction of the QOF.[42]

Although clinical indicators within the QOF have the potential to impact significantly on health (as measured by lives saved), the evidence linking QOF performance to measures of clinical performance suggest that at least some improvements predated the QOF. However, the rates of change of incentivised and non-incentivised activities appear to have diverged since its introduction.

Area-based inequalities

It has been estimated that 60% of the difference in mortality between deprived and affluent areas is due to conditions that are addressed in the QOF.[43] We have examined area-based variations and changes in practice performance on those QOF indicators that evidence suggests contribute to health gain or improvements in public health (SDO Project: 08/1716/207, 'Impact of QOF on GP practice, public health outcomes and health inequalities in England'). We explored the difference in performance between practices in Spearhead and non-Spearhead areas, and the association between the socio-economic status of the practices' population and its performance – controlling for practice characteristics known to affect performance, as well as other socio-economic characteristics.

Non-Spearhead practices slightly out-performed Spearhead practices on a subset of clinical indicators in both years. The improvements in Spearheads have been greater, so the gap in performance has narrowed. No difference in performance was observed among the most deprived practices between those in Spearhead and non-Spearhead areas.

The narrowing in performance between practices in Spearhead and non-Spearhead PCTs may have indirectly contributed to a reduction in area-based health inequalities, but the differences are small. The lack of difference between the most deprived practices in Spearhead and non-Spearhead PCTs suggests that area-based initiatives to tackle inequalities have not yet had an observable impact on practices deprived areas. As in previous studies, we found significant associations between QOF achievement and practice-level characteristics such as the number of GPs in the practice, country of GP education, caseload and personal medical services (PMS) status. However, the weak explanatory power of the model suggests that other factors may play a role in explaining variation in performance, e.g., aspects of practice organisation or other characteristics of the practice population.

CONCLUSIONS

Overall, the published evidence suggests that differences in performance between practices in deprived and non-deprived areas as measured by the QOF are narrowing. There is weak evidence to demonstrate the role of the QOF in reducing health inequalities. It is difficult to be certain whether improvements in performance represent a real change in clinical activity and therefore a commensurate improvement in health inequalities. It is equally plausible that the differences simply reflect differences in the organisational capacity of the practices, and their ability to monitor and report activities (as examined in Chapters 6 and 10). Given the weak explanatory power of the current models, it appears there are other non-observed factors that explain differences in performance as measured by the QOF. Although it is encouraging that the gap in performance between deprived and non-deprived practices, and between Spearhead and non-Spearhead areas, has narrowed, it is not yet clear that this has or will translate into reduced health inequalities.

Any reduction in health inequalities as a result of the QOF has been a positive side effect rather than an explicit objective. A recent Health Select Committee report on health inequalities recognised the role that the QOF can play and recommended that 'tackling health inequalities should be an explicit objective during annual QOF negotiations and that this objective should have measurable characteristics, which can be evaluated over time'.[44] As Campbell and Lester (Chapter 3) have described, the National Institute for Health and Clinical Excellence (NICE) is tasked with developing an independent and transparent process for reviewing new QOF indicators, which places particular emphasis on the cost effectiveness of QOF indicators.[45] NICE has signalled the importance of addressing health inequalities in the QOF by listing it as one of the eight criteria used to score potential topics.

Although NICE recognises the need for a greater focus on health inequalities within the QOF, it is not yet clear how this will be achieved as many of the major public health issues lack the evidence required by NICE for inclusion in the QOF. Many of the current indicators relate to clinical processes, which are easier to measure and for which there is available evidence. Outcomes, particularly those related to ill-health prevention, rely on factors such as patient adherence and wider socio-economic inputs.[46] Prevention-related indicators may take months or years to yield benefits. For example, the effects of increasing physical exercise beyond simple weight loss may take years to demonstrate. It is also difficult to assess whether a GP's actions are responsible for an individual's decision to change lifestyle behaviours such as increasing exercise or losing weight. As a result, some public health and prevention indicators may never be suitable for the QOF.

Even though other factors may influence the activities that general practices undertake to address health inequalities, the QOF provides a powerful set of financial incentives. It is therefore vital that the indicators selected and the weighting of points are, where possible, aligned to the objective of reducing health inequalities. First, a greater proportion of QOF indicators need to be linked directly to outcomes, e.g., quit rates for smoking, reduced emergency admissions for ambulatory care sensitive conditions. Second, thresholds within the QOF need to be set, so that there are sufficient incentives for proactive case finding, particularly in deprived areas where disease prevalence rates are higher. Finally, more work is needed to understand whether other incentives for staff working in primary care, both financial and non-financial, improve access for the hard to reach and those with greater healthcare needs. The challenge remains: how to ensure primary care plays its part in helping to turn the tide of health inequalities.

ACKNOWLEDGEMENTS

This chapter includes material from independent research commissioned by the National Institute for Health Research (NIHR) Service Delivery and Organisation (SDO) programme.

REFERENCES

1. Gillam S, Meads G. *Modernisation and the Future of General Practice.* London: King's Fund; 2001.
2. Department of Health. *Developing the Quality and Outcomes Framework: proposals for a new, independent process (consultation);* 2008. Available at: http://tinyurl.com/yc9geld
3. Department of Health. *Tackling Health Inequalities: 2006–08 policy and data update for the 2010 national target;* 2009. Available at: http://tinyurl.com/ylmc2v9
4. Ibid.
5. Health Inequalities Unit DoH. *Tackling Health Inequalities: 2006–08 policy and date update for the 2010 national target;* 2009. Available at: www.dh.gov.uk/publications
6. Ibid.
7. Ibid.
8. Healthcare Commission. *The Annual Health Check 2007/08.* London: Healthcare Commission; 2009.
9. Department of Health, 2009, op. cit.
10. Department of Health, 2009, op. cit.
11. Department of Health. *Tackling Health Inequalities: a programme for action;* 2003. Available at: http://tinyurl.com/26tros
12. The Marmot Review. *Fair Society, Healthy Lives;* 2010. Available at: www.ucl.ac.uk/gheg/marmotreview/Documents/finalreport/
13. Doran T. Delivery systems and mechanisms for reducing inequalities in both social determinants and health outcomes. *Final Report of Task Group 7, Part 3: Case study on an experiment in altering the system dynamic—the Quality and Outcomes Framework (QOF) initiative;* 2010. Available at: www.ucl.ac.uk/gheg/marmotreview
14. Ibid.
15. Doran T, Fullwood C, Gravelle H, *et al.* Pay-for-performance programmes in family practices in the United Kingdom. *N Engl J Med.* 2006; **355**(4): 375–84.
16. Ashworth M, Seed P, Armstrong D, *et al.* The relationship between social deprivation and the quality of primary care: a national survey using indicators from the UK Quality and Outcomes Framework. *Br J Gen Pract.* 2007; **57**(539): 441–8.
17. Doran T, Fullwood C, Kontopantelis E, *et al.* Effect of financial incentives on inequalities in the delivery of primary clinical care in England: analysis of clinical activity indicators for the Quality and Outcomes Framework. *Lancet.* 2008; **372**(9640): 728–36.
18. Ashworth M, Medina J, Morgan M. Effect of social deprivation on blood pressure monitoring and control in England: a survey of data from the Quality and Outcomes Framework. *BMJ.* 2008; **337**: a2030.
19. Sahota N, Hood A, Shankar A, *et al.* Developing performance indicators for primary care: Walsall's experience. *Br J Gen Pract.* 2008; **58**(557): 856–61.
20. Wang Y, O'Donnell CA, Mackay DF, *et al.* Practice size and quality attainment under the new GMS contract: a cross-sectional analysis. *Br J Gen Pract.* 2006; **56**(532): 830–5.
21. Ashworth M, Armstrong D. The relationship between general practice characteristics and quality of care: a national survey of quality indicators used in the UK Quality and Outcomes Framework, 2004–5. *BMC Fam Pract.* 2006; **7**: 68.

22. Doran, Fullwood, Kontopantelis, *et al.*, op. cit.
23. Saxena S, Car J, Eldred D, *et al.* Practice size, caseload, deprivation and quality of care of patients with coronary heart disease, hypertension and stroke in primary care: national cross-sectional study. *BMC Health Serv Res.* 2007; 7: 96.
24. Doran T, Fullwood C, Reeves D, *et al.* Exclusion of patients from pay-for-performance targets by English physicians. *N Engl J Med.* 2008; **359**: 274–84.
25. House of Commons: Health Committee. *Health Inequalities, Part 6: the role of the NHS in tackling health inequalities*. Third report of session 2008–09, Vol. I. Report No.: HC 286-I. London: TSO (The Stationery Office); 2009.
26. Department of Health. *Developing the Quality and Outcomes Framework: proposals for a new, independent process; consultation response and analysis*; 2009. Available at: http://tinyurl.com/ychag3r
27. Doran, op. cit.
28. Fleetcroft R, Cookson R. Do the incentive payments in the new NHS contract for primary care reflect likely population health gains. *J Health Serv Res Policy.* 2006; **11**(1): 27–31.
29. University of East Anglia, University of York. *Quality and Outcomes Framework*; 2008 [cited 5 May 2009]. Available at: http://tinyurl.com/dcu4e6
30. Ibid.
31. Bottle A, Millett C, Xie Y, *et al.* Quality of primary care and hospital admissions for diabetes mellitus in England. *J Ambul Care Manage.* 2008; **31**(3): 226–38.
32. Downing A, Rudge G, Cheng Y, *et al.* Do the UK government's new Quality and Outcomes Framework (QOF) scores adequately measure primary care performance? A cross-sectional survey of routine healthcare data. *BMC Health Serv Res.* 2007; **7**(1): 166.
33. Strong M, South G, Carlisle R. The UK Quality and Outcomes Framework pay-for-performance scheme and spirometry: rewarding quality or just quantity? A cross-sectional study in Rotherham, UK. *BMC Health Serv Res.* 2009; 9: 108.
34. Williams PH, de Lusignan S. Does a higher 'quality points' score mean better care in stroke? An audit of general practice medical records. *Inform Prim Care.* 2006; **14**(1): 29–40.
35. The Information Centre, NHS. *Time Series Analysis for 2001–2006 for Selected Clinical Indicators from the Quality and Outcomes Framework*. QRESEARCH; 2007.
36. Khunti K, Gadsby R, Millett C, *et al.* Quality of diabetes care in the UK: comparison of published quality-of-care reports with results of the Quality and Outcomes Framework for Diabetes. *Diabet Med.* 2007; **24**(12): 1436–41.
37. Crawley D, Ng A, Mainous AG, *et al.* Impact of pay for performance on quality of chronic disease management by social class group in England. *J R Soc Med.* 2009; **102**(3): 103–7.
38. Gulliford MC, Ashworth M, Robotham D, *et al.* Achievement of metabolic targets for diabetes by English primary care practices under a new system of incentives. *Diabet Med.* 2007; **24**(5): 505–11.
39. Alabbadi I, Crealey G, Turner K, *et al.* Statin prescribing in Northern Ireland and England pre and post introduction of the Quality and Outcomes Framework. *Pharm World Sci.* 2010; **32**(1): 43–51.
40. MacBride-Stewart SP, Elton R, Walley T. Do quality incentives change prescribing patterns in primary care? An observational study in Scotland. *Fam Pract.* 2008; **25**(1): 27–32.

41. Phillips LA, Donovan KL, Phillips AO. Renal quality outcomes framework and eGFR: impact on secondary care. *QJM*. 2009; **102**(6): 415–23.
42. The Marmot Review, op. cit.
43. House of Commons: Health Committee, op. cit.
44. Ibid.
45. Department of Health, 2008, op. cit.
46. Watts B, Lawrence R, Litaker D, *et al*. Quality of care by a hypertension expert: a cautionary tale for pay-for-performance approaches. *Qual Manag Health Care*. 2008; **17**(1): 35–46.

CHAPTER 6

'Smoke and mirrors'? Informatics opportunities and challenges

Maria Kordowicz and Mark Ashworth

SUMMARY

This chapter presents the informatics opportunities of the Quality and Outcomes Framework (QOF), while exploring the challenges this 'pay-for-performance' (P4P) initiative poses for capturing the quality of primary care. The successes of the QOF data systems are evaluated in light of the QOF's vulnerability to gaming and manipulation. Finally, the limitations of the QOF's use in research and as a public health improvement tool are examined.

Key points
- The QOF has provided a wealth of previously unavailable informatics opportunities to primary care.
- New data structures have been introduced to capture real-time data coding related to the QOF clinical indicators.
- Apparent improvements in care are due to better coding and recording of data.
- Exception reporting and lower targets limit improvements in outcomes.
- The opportunities are not without their limitations, which are linked to the QOF's vulnerability to the gaming of financial rewards for performance.

INTRODUCTION

The QOF has in many ways been a triumph. It is now hard to imagine consultations with patients and strategies for day-to-day practice management without the ever-present spectre of the QOF. Whether it is the QOF alerts appearing unbidden on the computer screen during patient consultations, motivational presentations about QOF targets within reach or the growing acceptance that the QOF strengthens the public health role of general practice, it seems that the QOF has succeeded in becoming part of the fabric of primary care.

The framework has brought with it new and improved data structures with previously unavailable opportunities for the collection, retrieval and application of general practice and patient information, with assumed potential for reducing public health inequalities. Nevertheless, there is a risk that the dominance of information from the QOF as the primary means of assessing general practice quality may lead to a misrepresentation of reality in which the policy smokescreen of performance in the QOF is considered synonymous with the quality of care that a patient receives in general practice.

The QOF required the implementation of information management and technology systems that were fit for the purpose of monitoring the performance of all general practices in England. This chapter explores important questions surrounding the shortcomings of informatics produced within a P4P framework.

QOF INFORMATICS AND SYSTEMS

Informatics in primary care is concerned with the management of data to enable specific interventions to be connected with changes in clinical indicators for a particular patient group. The implementation of new data structures to capture the coding of QOF clinical indicators saw a move away from unorganised data at general practice level to data processed in context. The QOF was not only a quality improvement initiative but also a tool for optimising the use of primary care information. The QOF holds data for 5 years covering +99.7% of registered patients in England.[1]

New information management and technology systems on this scale must be 'fit for purpose'. This is where the national quality management and analysis system (QMAS) came in. The purpose of QMAS was to collate QOF data, run practice system updates three times a year and provide feedback to practices about their performance against national QOF targets upon which payments were based. The National Health Service Connecting for Health website boldly states that QMAS allows for practices to be paid 'according to the quality of care they provide'. This implies – questionably – that high QOF scores are viewed as being synonymous with high quality care.[2]

Such a complex system needed to be fully functional during its first year to avoid payment failures for general practitioners (GPs). There were political risks in launching a computerised quality scoring structure linked to payments in the first year of the QOF. Had QMAS not translated quality points into payment accurately, the QOF could have been rejected by GPs. In the year following the QOF's inception, GPs were consistently paid in line with the new General Medical Services (GMS) contract rules. The integration of QMAS into primary care was hailed as a success.

A further information technology response following the introduction of QOF was the adaptation of in-practice systems and electronic patient records to allow for QMAS compatibility and more sensitive READ code searches year on year. The resulting software now provides prompts for clinicians to gather QOF-related data during a consultation and has entrenched the use of electronic templates for this purpose. It appears that this more methodical approach to patient consultations has been accepted by GPs and other primary care professionals.[3]

This improved infrastructure for primary care informatics has also yielded the largest national primary care database in the world. A discussion of the value and drawbacks of this in relation to research is given in the following sections.

QOF and research

Publicly available QOF data have provided researchers with a wealth of information at their fingertips. Before the QOF, researchers relied on the goodwill of the few practices open to taking part in research studies, which resulted in selection bias and participant fatigue. However, the use of QOF informatics as a research tool has drawbacks.

One limitation concerns the blurred distinction between audit and original research. Using routinely collated service, audit data in research requires a thorough consideration of consent and confidentiality. The QOF was designed solely for the purpose of monitoring care and identifying opportunities for service improvement by focusing on financial incentives in a particular domain. As QOF data are gathered purely for payment purposes, information about practice performance that is not linked to GMS contract financial rewards is omitted from the scheme. Researchers hoping to study GP consultation and diagnostic skills for instance have to look for data beyond those available through the QOF.

However, it is not just qualitative data that are lacking. The QOF informatics does not provide information about patient demographics, such as sex and age, within particular chronic disease groups. QOF data are presented in a way that does not allow for the modelling of relationships between the indicators across chronic disease domains, apart from smoking status and advice, which can be viewed across all disease categories. The lack of a cross-tabulation function does not allow for chronic disease multi-morbidity searching. One person who may have something to say about this is the patient who is called in for numerous reviews towards the end of the accounting year, instead of a single coordinated person-centred consultation. Naturally, this issue goes beyond limitations of the QOF for research and has implications for public health disease prevalence studies.

A further point concerns the research validity of QOF data. The prevalence of each of the 19 chronic diseases currently included in the QOF is not independently verified. There is some evidence for example of QOF coronary heart disease (CHD) underreporting as compared with self-reported census rates.[4] As such, a practice may simply have been ineffective in building up their disease registers. Patients who, for one reason or another, have not been coded or been incorrectly coded will not be on the disease register. The practice of exception reporting (*see* later) may exclude certain patients from the register again leading to selection bias.

This brings to light another important implication for the usefulness of QOF informatics in representing practice performance: self-evidently, there is an association between approaches to data recording and practice performance in the QOF. The key question is whether QOF performance merely reflects the data recording skills of a practice, rather than the quality of care it offers.

Better care or better recorded care?

Practices with more highly developed management infrastructures and a shared ethos of coding every possible QOF-related activity will inevitably have higher QOF scores at the end of the accounting year. Many apparent improvements in care amount to little more than increased conscientious coding. For example, a practice failing to reach the 90% target for retinopathy screening in diabetes mellitus (DM21) may find that this target is achievable simply by searching through scanned correspondence from the hospital diabetic clinic or local optometrist reporting retinopathy findings.

As Simon and Morton describe in Chapter 8, the practice will be making economic decisions based on workload, time and type of professional needed to reach the target. On this basis, a practice may make one of the three decisions. It may decide that it is not cost-effective to chase the final QOF point (DM21 is worth 5 points for achieving a 90% target) and remain below the top target. Or it may invest in additional data input staff to find and code missing clinical data. Or, and most expensively, it may invest in additional medical personnel to examine, say, an additional 10 patients with diabetes in order to gain all five available QOF points.

Better recording undoubtedly results in higher QOF points but may not represent better care. Equally, low-scoring practices may be less skilled at handling large data volumes and not necessarily be providing poorer care. It is possible that low-scoring practices display other domains of excellence not captured by the QOF, such as continuity of care, patient-centred consultation skills, diagnostic skills and care of illnesses not included in the QOF. Some commentators have described the QOF not so much as a P4P system, but a 'pay-for-reporting' system.[5] This clear link between methods for data recording and QOF performance, coupled with financial incentives for achieving high QOF scores may render the scheme vulnerable to data manipulation or gaming.

Gaming and P4P

With value for money and quality improvement as the main political drivers behind health policy development, the QOF P4P system was seen both as a means to make primary care more accountable to the public and a tool to incentivise improved quality of care. However, the introduction of financial incentives may motivate some healthcare professionals to manipulate data in order to increase QOF scores and therefore financial rewards.[6] Moreover, the public availability of QOF data stigmatises practices scoring poorly on the QOF and produces a means of ranking general practices. Gaming behaviours are further motivated by attempts to avoid such stigma.[7] Hood[8] describes three types of gaming presented in Table 6.1 with possible QOF applications.

Gaming is not unique to the QOF and is probably a feature of all P4P systems. The National Audit Office report on the 2004 new contract for GPs suggested that QOF income could be inappropriately boosted by deliberately removing patients for whom GPs may perhaps miss QOF targets from disease registers or by increasing levels of exception reporting.[9] In this vein, it has been suggested that exception reporting, although high in only a small proportion of practices, is the strongest predictor of practice achievement in the QOF.[10] There may well be more kudos to achieving high QOF scores for a small number of patients limited by exception reporting, than in gaining average scores across a larger and fuller chronic disease register with fewer exceptions.

On the other hand, the QOF provides financial incentives for increasing the number of patients recorded on a disease register, because the QMAS adjusts payments on the basis of disease prevalence. This may encourage the inclusion of patients with clinical measures on the cusp of diagnostic criteria on a particular chronic disease register. In other words, gaming may medicalise patients' problems placing them at a risk of unnecessary disease monitoring and inappropriate treatment.

Gaming may generate overlarge financial rewards for some practices but how widespread is it? Some have suggested that gaming is endemic, but a more balanced perspective emerged from the Centre of Health Economics, which concluded that

TABLE 6.1 Types of gaming and QOF opportunities

Type of gaming	Definition	QOF opportunities
Threshold effect	Reduction of performance to just what the target requires	Practices will still be rewarded financially for working to a certain percentage of the target, rather than meeting it for 100% of patients on a given register. Exception reporting so as to reduce workload
Ratchet effect	Underperformance to prevent target increase	Targets are set nationally and underperformance in single practices is unlikely to influence the level at which a target is set
Output distortion	Intentional manipulation of reported results	A spectrum running from selecting indicators for data entry that fits the target best, through to QOF fraud

practices could have treated 12.5% fewer patients without falling below upper QOF thresholds.[11] This suggests that practices have not produced a threshold-gaming effect, whereby the quantity and quality of work is reduced to the minimum needed to meet the target. In other words, general practices had overshot targets to a much larger extent than the likely level of exception reporting. Indeed Figure 6.1 shows a decrease in exception reporting nationally, across the last 4 years of QOF data (exception reporting rates were not available through QMAS for the year 2004/05).

Nevertheless, one of the challenges of the QOF remains how to tackle the potential for gaming, which is inherent in any P4P scheme. Although all general practices undergo an inspection-type visit annually by representatives from the primary care trust, these may be insufficient to detect evidence at case level of inappropriate exception reporting or exclusions from disease registers. Although inspection guidance makes a distinction between data manipulation due to error and by intention,[12] subtle levels of gaming may not be picked up and simple errors may be labelled as QOF fraud.

Inconsistencies in data entry within practices may be influenced by the lack of clear guidance on the methods for measuring and recording indicators, rather than fraudulent activity. For instance, a blood pressure reading in a patient's electronic notes may be the 'best' of three measurements taken in a consultation, the average of readings taken on separate occasions or even the reading that is closest to the target entered electronically from paper notes by the practice administrator. This is further compounded by the fact that target levels recommended by the GMS contract differ from those promoted by National Institute for Health and Clinical Excellence (NICE) and the British Hypertension Society. This has led some commentators to state that defining QOF targets without clear guidance is 'largely meaningless'.[13] What looks like fraudulent data recording may simply be the result of clustering due to unclear methodological guidance. It is unlikely that P4P will ever produce normally distributed epidemiological data, yet PCT assessors are advised to investigate clustering that appears not to be the result of 'energetic treatment'.[14]

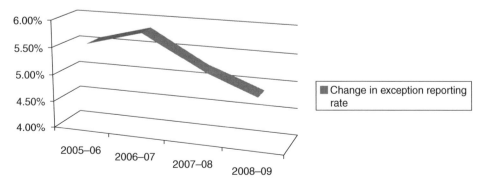

FIGURE 6.1 National QOF exception reporting rates

The notion of the healthcare professional gaming data in order to achieve financial gain is likely to be an oversimplification. Studies have shown that unless external incentives such as payments for performance appeal to the professional values of the individual concerned, they paradoxically reduce performance.[15] Professionalism as a driver of quality is in danger of being ignored by the QOF. However, it is a sense of professionalism, the accumulation of a body of specialist knowledge and wisdom placed at the service of society, and a public service ethos that probably motivate GPs more in the long term. It is hard to see how any P4P system could reward the components of professionalism expounded by Downie such as honesty, fairness and conduct, which is legal, ethical and having legitimate authority.[16]

However, there can be no doubt that debates concerning gaming behaviours in general practice do not hold the same significance for patient care as the key question of whether or not the QOF and QOF informatics have led to tangible improvements in the nation's health.

Illusory public health gains?

There is no doubt that the QOF has contributed to overall improvements in quality and gains in 'intermediate outcomes' such as blood pressure and cholesterol control. However, the successes of the QOF have been tempered by concerns that some of these achievements might not be as substantial as they appear to be.

The quality of chronic disease management proved to be far higher than was thought at the time the QOF was introduced. The Department of Health based pay calculations on an expected QOF score of 750 at the end of the first year (2004/05). In fact, the 8600 practices in England had a mean QOF score of 958.7 (out of a maximum possible score of 1050 points), which represented 91.3% of available points.[17] Two hundred twenty-two (2.6%) of these practices achieved the maximum score. In spite of several annual revisions to the QOF, revising targets upwards and adding indicators, the 2008/09 mean QOF score achievement was 954.2 of available points (the maximum is currently 1000 points) with 2.0% of practices achieving the maximum score (*see* Figure 6.2).[18]

These scoring gains have also translated into public health gains, albeit on a rather piecemeal basis. In an evaluation of the QOF in its original incarnation, Fleetcroft and Cookson, concluded that there was 'no relationship between pay and health gain', at least for the eight public health and preventative interventions, which were included in their study.[19] This is unsurprising, given that the levels of financial reward were based on estimates of predicted GP workload. However, for the QOF to continue being generously funded, it has to demonstrate that it is money well spent in terms of health gains.

The weighting of QOF points, the result of annual haggling over GP pay, continues to be driven by the assumed workload attached to achieving each indicator and not the likely benefit to patients. Thus, the indicator DM23 (50% achievement of

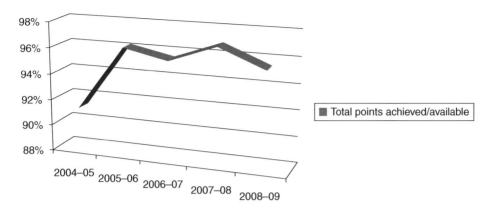

FIGURE 6.2 QOF scores nationally 2004/09 as a percentage of total points achieved out of the total available

an HbA1c target for diabetics of 7.0 or less) is awarded 17 points, whereas DM18 (influenza vaccination target of 85% for diabetics) attracts just 3 points. Moreover, many of the public health indicators within the QOF such as blood pressure, cholesterol and HbA1c control were improving before its inception. Nevertheless, there has been evidence of further public health gain with substantial improvements in, for instance, the management of diabetes and control of cardiovascular risk factors in patients with diabetes.[20]

A further public health success has been the drive to reduce health inequalities. The differences in QOF achievement between deprived and prosperous areas have been small and, over time, there is evidence that these differences have diminished.[21] The narrowing of target differences between rich and poor communities has been part of an overall trend of improved performance with somewhat greater improvements seen in more deprived communities (*see* Chapters 4 and 5).[22]

Factors limiting improvements from the QOF

One reason for questioning the success of P4P in its incarnation as the QOF is that three technical features of the QOF may have diminished the reach of performance targets.

First, the process of 'exception reporting' allows certain patients, deemed 'unsuitable', to be excluded from the overall target for patients registered at the practice. Patients may understandably be excluded if they are terminally ill or if they do not agree (after three written requests) to attend an appointment at the surgery for the management of their chronic disease. Non-attenders will be excluded and the public health effectiveness of population targets will be reduced. The overall exception reporting rate for 2008/09 was 6.88% for indicators measuring an outcome and 1.70% for indicators measuring a process. So, on average, almost 7% of patients in England are excluded from public health targets such as achievement of a serum cholesterol of <5 mmol/L.

Second, the targets are not set at 100% – again understandable, given the practical difficulties of achieving clinical targets. These targets are rarely achieved in research trial conditions, let alone in routine practice. However, targets set at 70% for blood pressure control or cholesterol control in CHD6 and CHD8 further exclude 30% of patients from these public health targets. Thus in combination with exception reporting, targets set below 100% may shift the focus of the practice away from harder to reach patients, in exchange for more efficient achievement of results.

The success of the QOF may be tempered in other respects. Performance may have improved in domains covered by performance indicators but remain static in areas, such as rheumatological and gastrointestinal disease, out of the financial spotlight. Increasingly, the proposals for strengthening the QOF are focusing on aligning the indicators and the associated QOF points with public health gains. With NICE taking overall responsibility for QOF development, the QOF is expected to develop in accordance with NICE guidelines and favour cost-effective public health interventions (*see* Chapter 3). Nevertheless, there are suggestions that performance has now reached a ceiling in some areas and that other approaches are needed to coax further improvements.

Another potential approach to quality improvement could be greater inclusion of feedback from patients. Before 2008, GPs simply gave out questionnaires to a selection of patients, and 'patient experience' points were awarded for having completed a survey and reflected on the results of these surveys. Since then, a more rigorous approach has been adopted with independent patient surveys conducted by polling organisations. GPs are now rewarded on the basis of responses to two questions about time taken to access an appropriate health professional (PE7 and PE8). The questions asked have been criticised as being politically driven and not representative of patients' needs; they do not ask about the consultation or perceived standards of care. One unintended consequence is that less satisfied responses from patients in deprived communities could result in less funding being directed toward practices serving populations with higher healthcare needs. However, the inclusion of these indicators does mark the incorporation of the patient 'voice' within QOF informatics.[23]

CONCLUSIONS

So is the QOF all smoke and mirrors, or has it produced advances in informatics that outweigh its limitations? There is no doubt that the QOF has brought a wealth of coherent primary care data that were previously unobtainable. Data used to provide performance monitoring information for general practices can be set against targets determined by the GMS contract and are now widely available. So too is information that contributes to identifying potential public health inequalities. However, the key lies in recognising the limits of how QOF informatics should be used. Bold statements about the QOF's power to raise and sustain the quality of patient care ignore the subtleties of gaming behaviours in the face of financial rewards.

The QOF represents only a snapshot of the day-to-day work of general practices in England. The underlying essence of good primary care lies in subjective notions of rapport, interpersonal skills, compassion and professionalism, which are unlikely ever to be fully captured through P4P initiatives. QOF informatics may therefore have illusory effects that detract from grounding quality improvement in the reality of patient experience. Nevertheless, the QOF has emerged as one part of a multifaceted approach to embed high quality care into routine practice.

REFERENCES

1. The Quality and Outcomes Framework. *The Health and Social Care Information Centre.* Leeds: The NHS Information Centre; 2009. Available at: www.qof.ic.nhs.uk/ (accessed 12 March 2010).
2. NHS Connecting for Health. *What is QMAS?* 2010. Available at: www.connecting forhealth.nhs.uk/systemsandservices/gpsupport/qmas (accessed 12 March 2010).
3. McDonald R, Harrison S, Checkland K. Incentives and control in primary healthcare: findings from English pay-for-performance case studies. *J Health Org Manag.* 2008; **22**(1): 48–62.
4. Martin D, Wright J. Disease prevalence in the English population: a comparison of primary care registers and prevalence models. *Sos Sci Med.* 2009; **68**: 266–74.
5. Lester H. The UK Quality and Outcomes Framework. *BMJ.* 2008; **337**: a2095.
6. Mangin D, Toop L. The Quality and Outcomes Framework: what have you done to yourselves? *Br J Gen Pract.* 2007; **57**(539): 435–7.
7. Lilford R, Mohammed MA, Spiegelhalter D, *et al.* Use and misuse of process and outcome data in managing performance of acute medical care: avoiding institutional stigma. *Lancet.* 2004; **363**(9415): 1147–54.
8. Hood C. Gaming in targetworld: the targets approach to managing British public services. *Pub Adm Rev.* 2006; **66**(4): 515–21.
9. National Audit Office. *NHS Pay Modernisation: new contracts for general practice services in England;* 2008. Available at: www.nao.org.uk/publications/0708/new_ contracts_for_general_prac.aspx (accessed 12 March 2010).
10. Doran T, Fullwood C, Gravelle H, *et al.* Pay-for-performance programs in family practices in the United Kingdom. *New Engl J Med.* 2006; **355**(4): 375–84.
11. Centre for Health Economics. *Doctor Behaviour Under a Pay for Performance Contract: evidence from the Quality and Outcomes Framework.* York: Centre for Health Economics; 2007. Available at: www.york.ac.uk/inst/che/pdf/rp28.pdf (accessed 12 March 2010).
12. NHS Employers. *Establishing Accuracy in QOF Data: A PCT assessors guide;* 2005. Available at www.connectingforhealth.nhs.uk/systemsandservices/gpsupport/qof/ docs/establishing_accuracy_in_qof_data.pdf (accessed 12 March 2010).
13. Manning G, Brooks A, Slinn B, *et al.* Assessing blood pressure control in patients treated for hypertension: comparing different measurements and targets. *Br J Gen Pract.* 2006; **56**(526): 375–7.

14. NHS Employers, op. cit.

15. Deci E, Koestner R, Ryan R. A meta-analytic review of experiments examining the effects of extrinsic rewards on intrinsic motivation. *Psychol Bull.* 1999; **125**(6): 692–700.

16. Downie R. Professions and professionalism. *J Philos Educ.* 1990; **24**: 147–59.

17. The Quality and Outcomes Framework, op. cit.

18. Ibid.

19. Fleetcroft R, Cookson R. Do the incentive payments in the new NHS contract for primary care reflect likely population health gains? *J Health Serv Res Policy.* 2006; **11**: 27–31.

20. Millett C, Saxena S, Ng A, *et al.* Socio-economic status, ethnicity and diabetes management: an analysis of time trends using the health survey for England. *J Public Health.* 2007; **29**: 413–19.

21. Ashworth M, Medina J, Morgan M. Effect of social deprivation on blood pressure monitoring and control in England: a survey of data from the Quality and Outcomes Framework. *BMJ.* 2008; **337**: a2030.

22. Lester H. The UK Quality and Outcomes Framework. *BMJ.* 2008; **337**: a2095.

23. Roland M, Elliott M, Lyratzopoulos G, *et al.* Reliability of patient responses in pay for performance schemes: analysis of national General Practitioner Patient Survey data in England. *BMJ.* 2009; **339**: b3851.

CHAPTER 7

The impact of the QOF on practice organisation and service delivery

Kath Checkland and Stephen Harrison

SUMMARY

In this chapter, we report the findings of two linked qualitative case studies in England and Scotland, which used interviews and observation to investigate in depth the impact of the Quality and Outcomes Framework (QOF) on practice organisation and service delivery in four general medical practices. A number of significant changes to practice organisation and service delivery were observed including: changes to practice organisational structures, an increased role for information technology, a move towards a more biomedical form of medical care and changes to roles and relationships including the introduction of internal peer review and surveillance. Despite this, the practices maintained a narrative of 'no change', arguing that they had 'fitted QOF in' to their routines with little trouble. We discuss the wider implications of these findings.

Key points

- All the practices that we studied had changed their structures and organisation in response to the new contract.
- Changes included employing additional staff, changing the roles of existing staff, and creating internal 'QOF teams', who carried responsibility for aspects of the framework.
- We found an increased role for information technology, with an emphasis on the use of structured data-collection templates.
- We found that practices had moved towards providing a more biomedical form of care.

- Despite what seemed to be quite significant changes, we found that practices maintained a narrative of 'no change' when discussing the new contract.

INTRODUCTION

Earlier chapters have described the development and implementation of the Quality and Outcomes Framework (QOF) in UK general practice. Meeting the evolving quality standards that the QOF embodies is not only an exercise in patient care by individuals (prescribing the right drugs and responding appropriately to test results outside the required range) but also requires collective activity within practices. Call and recall systems, accurate computerised records, clear allocation of responsibilities and frequent audits of achievement are all required to maximise performance against the targets, and success has been generally well rewarded at the practice level, with practice incomes increasing significantly, at least initially.[1]

Studies of achievement of QOF targets, and before/after comparisons of care can tell us something about the outcomes of this collective activity,[2] but they tell us little about the impact on practices as a whole or on the overall nature of the care that practices provide.

This chapter summarises the results of two linked qualitative studies of the impact of the QOF on four general medical practices across the United Kingdom (in England and Scotland). Following a brief summary of the research, the main findings of the studies are presented under four headings, each accompanied by a brief analytical commentary. The concluding section discusses the surprising finding that practice staff largely saw the major changes resulting from the QOF as relatively insignificant in terms of the nature of general medical practice.

THE RESEARCH

The evidence presented here derives from the results of two linked ethnographic case studies of the new contract, involving two practices in England and two in Scotland. The methods are described in more detail elsewhere.[3] Data collection included observation and interviews, and took place over approximately 5 months in 2006. This period covered the introduction of the new QOF indicators for depression and kidney disease. A qualitative approach was adopted because we were interested in the fine-grained detail of practice responses to the QOF. Murphy *et al.*[4] suggest that qualitative methods are particularly useful: '...for studying socially meaningful behaviour, holistically, in context and with due attention to the dynamic processual aspects of social events and interactions'. Furthermore, by observing practice activity, both formally in meetings and informally in reception areas, etc., we were able to go beyond participants' accounts of what they did and observe directly from the processes and interactions that

TABLE 7.1 Practice characteristics

	Medium practice	*Big practice*	*Family practice*	*Modern practice*
List size	7900	12 000	4870	8000 increasing to 9000 during the study
Setting	English suburban, high numbers of families	English inner city, deprived population	Scottish middle-sized university town, high proportion of students and the elders	Scottish medium-sized town, deprived population
Doctors	Four partners	Seven partners, two salaried GPs	Three partners	Six partners, two salaried GPs
Nurses	Three nurse practitioners, one practice nurse, one healthcare assistant	Two nurse practitioner, three 'chronic disease' nurses, two healthcare assistants	Three practice nurses, one healthcare assistant	Three practice nurses, two healthcare assistants
Self-identification	Public health focus	Large, but holistic	Traditional 'family doctors'	Modern and business-like

determine overall practice responses to change. The characteristics of the four practices are listed in Table 7.1.

The results of studies such as those described here cannot be said to be 'representative' in the statistical sense and are inevitably small in scale because of the time required to collect and analyse detailed observational data. However, it was striking how similar the trajectories of change that we observed were in a set of practices that had little in common either in the way that they were organised or in the ways in which they identified themselves. This suggests that, although caution must be employed, our findings are unlikely to apply only to a narrow subset of practices. A number of papers have been published reporting different aspects of these results, some of which report results from both studies[5,6,7] and some based solely upon the English practices.[8,9,10,11] This paper summarises evidence from both sets of papers.

THE IMPACT ON PRACTICE ORGANISATION

General practices in the United Kingdom have become ever more complex organisations over the past decades, with increasing numbers of both clinical and other staff employed.[12] They face increasing managerial challenges.[13,14] Research has demonstrated that it is not enough simply to think about practices as collections of individual general practitioners (GPs): while the views and attitudes of individual doctors may be interesting, the response of practices to change is an interactive outcome within the organisation as a whole.[15] All the practices that we studied had changed their modes of operation in response to the QOF. Although the details were different in each practice, in general, this involved an increase in the number of administrative staff, including those with responsibility for information technology (IT). In addition, three of the four practices recruited extra healthcare assistants, in one case promoting existing administrative staff to these positions. This particular practice had not recruited any additional qualified nurses, but the other three had done so. In all cases, this represented an overall increase in practice expenses, which tended to offset the financial gains resulting from the new contract. All of the practices had set up a formal or informal internal 'QOF team', who were responsible for administering the QOF process, ensuring systems were in place to collect the necessary data, checking audits to ensure targets were being met and setting up call and recall systems to send for patients. In some practices, these responsibilities were diffused, with individual staff members responsible for different clinical areas (e.g., nurses with diabetes experience responsible for diabetic indicators), whereas in others a single staff member assumed overall responsibility for the whole range of QOF work. Internal hierarchies developed with, e.g., *Medium* practice promoting three receptionists to form the 'IT team', who not only had higher status than their reception colleagues but were also involved at a very early stage in decision-making about how to address new QOF targets. Managers' roles gained in importance, as they assumed responsibility for delivering the 500 points devoted to 'managerial' domains and for overseeing the achievement in the clinical domains. Many of the practices had set up new clinics for patients with chronic diseases, and in all the study sites, while attempts were made to minimise duplication, patients with more than one chronic disease were subject to multiple recalls to attend the practice.

THE ROLE OF IT

Attainment of QOF targets is assessed by the automatic extraction of data from practice computer systems on a certain date each year; therefore, data collection in general practice has assumed a greater importance than ever before. The official discourse surrounding the computerisation of medical records is unremittingly positive, claiming that benefits include: convenience and confidence (for patients), integration of care, improving outcomes, better use of evidence, better audit and improved efficiency.[16] Much of the medical informatics literature views the electronic record as a neutral recording device, whose benefits or disbenefits depend solely upon the efficiency with which it does the job for which it is designed.[17,18,19,20] However, there is a more critical sociological literature that points out that electronic records shape not only the way in which medical care is conceived of and delivered but also the nature of the host organisation and the work within that organisation.[21,22] Thus, who is allowed to enter data into a record is both shaped by and will shape the organisational hierarchy. Similarly, a record that only allows the recording of 'yes/no' factual data that can be coded into categories will tend to crowd out and devalue softer, more nuanced contextual information.[23] Not only will a structured record shape the way a job is performed day to day but also it becomes part of the definition of the nature of that job in the longer term.[24] In all of our practices, data recording via templates had become the norm. These templates act both to define the nature of the work required by acting as 'prompts', and to discourage staff from recording un-coded information that is not important for the QOF process.[25] As a result, a nuanced clinical encounter may be reduced to a series of 'yes/no' answers on a template. Furthermore, we found evidence that for new, less experienced staff, the existing templates were used as training devices: 'doing a cardiovascular check' became 'filling in the cardiovascular disease template'. The data-collection templates therefore not only structured and shaped clinician–patient encounters in the here-and-now but also their use as training devices ensured that the current definition of the nature of the job would be perpetuated into the future. Finally, we found that the increased use of IT altered practice structures and roles in more subtle ways. In *Medium* practice, e.g., 'writing the templates' and 'organising the recall systems' became important roles that altered existing power relationships (*see* Box 7.1).

Box 7.1 New roles and power relationships

So the one deal is that nobody messes with the due diary dates, recall systems or any clinical review system without prior discussion. They mustn't suspend or change a due diary date, or do anything if they don't understand what they are fiddling with. [Doctor 1, Medium]

In *Big* practice, having responsibility for checking the IT system to look for patients not meeting QOF targets gave the nurses (and doctors) concerned the legitimacy to 'chase' their colleagues by, e.g., sending notes to request that certain checks are made when patients attend for routine consultations. In *Medium* practice, there was a newly constituted 'IT team'. When new clinical indicators were issued in April 2006, rather than being discussed first by the doctors in order to discuss their clinical merits/demerits, the first meetings were held between the partner with QOF responsibilities and the IT team. Only once this group had produced an implementation plan was there any discussion with the wider team. In this way, new indicators were configured as a technical problem requiring an IT solution, rather than as a clinical problem requiring a clinical response by the doctors.

In summary, therefore, our studies demonstrated that the QOF and its associated IT requirements acted to configure a patient whose complaints were categorised into a series of clinical codes, a clinical encounter that followed a pre-determined pattern and a practice structure that privileged those with IT access and roles.

IMPACT ON THE CLINICAL ENCOUNTER AND ON THE NATURE OF MEDICAL CARE

The development of general practice as an academic specialty was, in part, founded upon opposition to the dominance of hospital medicine in the 1950s and 1960s. The latter was said to be characterised by what is now generally called the 'biomedical model',[26,27] in which the human body is seen as a host for disease, and therapeutic interventions were directed at the disease rather than the individual. In contrast, the *Royal College of General Practitioners* 1972 publication, *The Future General Practitioner* emphasises the role of GPs as being concerned with 'the patient's total experience of illness',[28] and coined the term 'patient-centred practice'.[29] Patient-centred care has remained a central concern of GPs,[30] though definitions of what is meant by patient-centred care are not always clear, and may not have necessarily been reflected in clinical practice.[31] Against this background, GPs in the United Kingdom have, along with their hospital counterparts, been encouraged to engage with the notion of 'evidence-based medicine' (EBM). The original proponents of this approach emphasised the integration of population evidence from randomised controlled trials with the unique personal preferences and health state of the individual[32] in a way that is entirely compatible with a 'patient-centred' approach. However, Harrison[33] has argued that in the UK National Health Service (NHS), this 'critical appraisal' model has been overtaken by 'scientific-bureaucratic medicine', i.e., the translation of research evidence into 'clinical guidelines' for the more or less routine application to classes of patients, defined according to their disease category. The documentation surrounding the QOF emphasises its underlying evidence-base,[34,35] and it can be argued that it represents a biomedical model of medical care, implemented by paying doctors to conform.

Thus, the very nature of the QOF suggests a biomedical approach to medical practice, and in our studies, we found that changes had been made that would result in patients receiving a more biomedical, less patient-centred form of care.[36] For example, in two of our practices non-attendance for required QOF checks was not accepted as a legitimate expression of dissent; patients who failed to attend in response to a number of letters would be visited at home (*see* Box 7.2).

Box 7.2 The biomedical approach to medical practice

So we have got, we have got the true house-bounds, but if there are other people who are ill with conditions who for whatever reason won't, or don't come in eventually a trained nurse and an auxiliary will go out and do it…so there's no escape. [Doctor 1, Medium]

Moreover, participants acknowledged that their consultations had become more 'biomedical', with an additional QOF-related agenda running alongside the patient's own agenda. Thus, e.g., reminder systems were set up so that when patients attended for unrelated problems, the doctors/nurses would be reminded to weigh them, take their blood pressures or check their urine. Although in many cases this would be unproblematic, our participants acknowledged that it could generate awkwardness, particularly if the data required were not related to the presenting problem in a particular consultation. Finally, it was clear that care within our practices had become more dependent upon pharmacological approaches to treatment. For example, the QOF requires blood pressure to be controlled within a certain period of time after diagnosis. Non-pharmacological measures may take time to work, and we found an increased tendency to treat early with tablets (*see* Box 7.3).

Box 7.3 Dependence upon pharmacological approaches to treatment

Some patients will come to you and they'll plead with you, 'please don't give me any tablets, I'll bring my blood pressure down, I'll do everything. I'll bring it down', and again they're not horrendously high, they're like say 140/90 or whatever…but we're saying to them 'well, look we've checked it three times now and it remains raised, you're clinically classed as hypertensive, we follow these guidelines and this is what we should be doing with you'. [Nurse practitioner, Medium]

Despite this evidence of a move towards a more biomedical approach, all of our participants claimed that they still were able to practice 'holistic' (a whole person approach to) medicine. Careful analysis of these claims to holism suggested that they rested upon the somewhat slippery definitions of 'holism' that exist. Thus, we found claims to holism variously based upon: a metaphorical 'protected space' within the consultation; an ideal of complexity claiming that doctors continued to treat 'complex' patients while their nursing colleagues dealt with routine QOF-related work; and the ability of doctors to maintain an 'overview' of patient care, even if they were not personally involved.

In summary, the QOF embodies a notion of medical care that is essentially biomedical in approach. In our study practices, this more biomedical approach had been adopted and had led to changes in the way that patients were treated within the practices. However, the doctors in our study seemed unaware of this change, using the ill-defined nature of 'holism' to continue to make rhetorical claims to be providing a patient-centred model of care.

CHANGING ROLES AND 'RESTRATIFICATION'

Before 1990, as long as he/she were conscientious and avoided complaints, what an individual doctor did in his or her own consulting room had no impact on the income of the practice as a whole. Health promotion clinics and immunisation targets made some impact in the early 1990s, and the advent of local medical audit advisory groups[37] introduced a generation of GPs to the notion of auditing performance. Achievement of QOF maximum scores, however, requires the actions of individuals to be scrutinised, and the use of computer monitoring systems makes consulting-room behaviour visible to all, thereby introducing collective responsibility into general practice on a scale not seen before.

In all of our study practices, we found subtle but important changes in roles and in boundaries between roles. Clinical staff fell into two groups: those responsible for ensuring that QOF targets were met, and those who were not. In one of our practices, these two groups identified themselves as 'chasers' and 'chased', and in all practices, mechanisms had been set up for monitoring achievement against the targets. Thus, in *Big* practice, responsibility for QOF targets was devolved down to individual clinical staff, including both doctors and nurses. Those responsible for a particular target would chase their colleagues by sending electronic notes and reminders (*see* Box 7.4).

Box 7.4 Changing roles and restratification

Every day I come in I check [performance]…I'm a chaser…if you're a chaser you have to chase yourself though. 'Cos you've no credibility if you don't deliver. [GP partner ID 16 Big].

Despite the practice initially identifying themselves as quite open and democratic in their management processes, by the end of the study period an internal 'management group' had been set up, and 'naming and shaming' of those seen to be 'not pulling their weight' with regard to QOF targets took place. In *Medium* and *Family* practices, one of the partners took responsibility for all the QOF targets, sending reminders to colleagues. There was a perception by those without formal QOF responsibilities that they might be 'told off' if they failed to comply. In *Modern* practice, naming and shaming took place at a practice meeting, but interestingly, it was largely the nurses who were subject to this process. The manager reported that he would approach the doctors individually about their QOF performance rather than naming them in public.

Thus, we found that new distinctions had grown up within practices between those who carried responsibility for QOF targets and those who did not; these groups can be conveniently labelled chasers and chased. Freidson drew attention to what has been subsequently called restratification between groups of physicians,[38] arguing that a new 'knowledge elite' had grown up, who were responsible for setting the agenda to be followed by what could be called 'rank and file' physicians. The changes that we observed suggest that the QOF has generated a new form of restratification within UK general practice, with some clinicians (both doctors and nurses) involved in surveillance of their colleagues. Freidson suggested that restratification such as this would threaten the solidarity of the professional group as a whole. In our study, by contrast, we found that, whereas some GPs expressed reservations about being chased and about the substantive content of some of the targets, there was little real dissent. Indeed, our study of the QOF, in combination with a later study of practice-based commissioning suggests that there may be new norms developing in UK general practice, in which peer review and surveillance are regarded as legitimate and indeed desirable.[39]

CHANGE BUT 'NO CHANGE'

The two studies discussed here demonstrated a number of changes that have occurred as a result of the QOF: practice structures, roles and processes have changed; increased use of IT has had an impact on the nature of consultations; the QOF itself has enacted a more biomedical approach to patient care; and the contract has legitimised internal peer review and surveillance. Despite these significant changes, all four practices that we studied offered us a narrative of 'no change'. Each practice had a clear, dominant 'story' about itself that 'explained' the approach taken to general practice work and organisation, the values underpinning this approach and their expectations of future developments.[40] The existence of such 'organisational stories', which act as repositories of organisational memory, determinants of organisational identity and as resources for both the socialisation of new organisational members and the presentation of the organisation to the outside world, is well recognised in the management literature.[41] These stories differed significantly between our study practices, ranging from the self-consciously 'small and traditional' *Family* practice, who described themselves as a 'dying breed', to the business-like *Modern* practice, which referred to 'customers' rather than patients. During the study, these four very different practices were all observed making changes that brought them closer together in structure, organisation and in the type of care that was offered. Despite this, they all maintained a rhetorical stance that there had been 'no real change' in response to the QOF (*see* Box 7.5).

Box 7.5 Convergence in organisation

All I think QOF did was make it a bit more organised and that. I don't think it was anything new. [GP4, Modern]

We were told that 'we were doing it already' or that the additional work had easily been 'fitted in' alongside their usual work. The narratives that underpinned their identities remained intact, despite an increasing discrepancy between the stories told and the reality on the ground. Our practices seemed to be aware neither of this discrepancy nor of the magnitude or potential impact of the changes that were occurring. It would seem from these two studies that the QOF has been construed by UK general practices as a technical problem, which has been efficiently solved.

From a wider social science perspective, the changes in practice organisation that we have observed can be been as part of a more general trend towards what we term the 'commodification' of healthcare in the NHS. This concept originally derives from a Marxist analysis of the treatment of goods and services as a means of exchange. In the current context, we distinguish between literal and conceptual commodification.[42] Literal commodification signifies the treatment of some good or service as if produced for the purpose of exchange, rather than simply for consumption[43]; its antonym 'decommodification' signifies the removal of a good or service from the market,[44] as is the case with NHS healthcare. It is clear from this description that a system such as that in the United Kingdom, in which care is not provided on a fee-for-service basis cannot be said to be literally commodified. However, conceptual commodification refers to the conceptualisation of the outputs of medical work in a standardised manner, in order to enable external control, and it is this idea that we argue has relevance here. This can be clarified by considering an ideal, typical representation of a doctor/patient relationship. As discussed earlier, GPs in the United Kingdom remain rhetorically wedded to an ideal of holistic care, in which medical care provided to patients is both 'co-produced' (i.e., results from interaction between the doctor's reaction to the patient's account of their problem and the patient's reaction to the doctor's diagnosis and prescribed treatment) and 'emergent' in the sense that therapy is decided upon and modified over time, depending on the patient's personal (psychological and social) and clinical responses to initial tests and treatment. Although external agents such as governments or insurers may exert indirect controls on this process through such devices as licensing and accreditation arrangements or pharmaceutical formularies, this co-production model of the medical relationship is difficult for an external agent to control directly, simply because each patient is unique and there is, therefore, no conceptual 'currency' in which to express what the doctor is required to do or to measure their workload. Conceptual commodification addresses this lacuna in external controllability by conceptualising the output of the medical labour process in a standardized manner. One manifestation of conceptual commodification that has become internationally ubiquitous in the healthcare field is the 'casemix' measure, originally developed in the United States as the diagnosis-related group and subsequently in the United Kingdom as the healthcare resource group (HRG). Such measures aim to categorize healthcare interventions into groups each of which is both clinically similar and uses the same unit amount of resource. Thus, the individualised doctor–patient interaction that generates a specific and unique management plan is replaced by a series of predefined routine treatments for defined categories of patients. Combined, for instance, with clinical guidelines and micro-economic analyses, casemix measures can then be used to form the basis of more complex but at the same time more routinised systems of 'managed care', 'disease management' and 'patient pathways'. Such conceptual commodification thus makes medical care more controllable by management. However, it can also facilitate literal commodification through large-scale competitive exchange, by allowing standardized product descriptions and prices. HRGs are increasingly employed as the basis of 'payment-by-results' relationships between NHS primary care trusts and secondary care providers, with each casemix classification carrying a nationally specified financial 'tariff'.

CONCLUSIONS

The QOF provides a manifestation of conceptual commodification that, unlike casemix measures, is currently unique to the United Kingdom (although international interest suggests that the approach might be adopted elsewhere). Our observations about the effect of the QOF on aspects of general practice organisation can also be construed as confirming its commodifying effects. First, the QOF itself codifies the work required for GPs and their staff, a process that is reinforced by some aspects of IT usage that we observed, notably the use of consultation 'templates' and the 'ticking of boxes' to signify completion of the specified tasks. Second, the QOF requires the aggregation of required elements of work in order to produce an overall score for the practice, a process that is reinforced by the use of 'population manager' software in order to track aggregate achievement almost in real time. Third, organisational efforts are redirected towards QOF achievement, with a wide range of practice staff, from partners and salaried GPs to nurses, healthcare assistants and receptionists, effectively co-opted into managerial tasks. Fourth, and underpinning all these changes, is the 'biomedical model', its intellectual dominance reinforced by the QOF. The sociological significance of these observations is potentially considerable. From one perspective, the QOF represents a triumph of medical professional power and dominance. The QOF reinforces longstanding medical world views and medical power over patients, without challenging GP perceptions of 'holism' and patient-centred practice, and in the process allowing those GPs (the majority) who are owners or part owners of general medical practices to increase their earnings.

From another perspective, however, the QOF may constitute a significant inroad into medical power: 'an unprecedented system of central control and external surveillance' as one commentator described it.[45] The irony is that this control and surveillance is facilitated by the biomedical model whose key assumptions are not unique to medicine but, crucially, are shared with those of management.[46] The biomedical model is in many respects a surgical model of ill health in the sense that it assumes potentially tangible and/or visible physical lesions as the cause of disease.[47,48] This effectively focuses medical attention on what two or more sufferers have in common (they become cases of a more general disease category), and away from the uniqueness of individual patients. Specifically, the assumption that ill health can be attributed to specific causes that have little to do with social or psychological contexts allows patients to be standardized, categorized and allocated to specific protocols or pathways. Moreover, the assumption that cases within a category are fundamentally homogeneous allows the ready application of the everyday tools of management; it permits the production and producers of 'cases' to be controlled bureaucratically and managerially. The primary result of conceptual commodification is that the occupiers of managerial roles are more easily able to control medical work.

Of course, such developments have not occurred in an ideational vacuum; the widespread international use of casemix measures has already been noted. Similar reductivist and managerialist ideas can be discerned in the manner in which EBM has been approached in the United Kingdom. In scientific-bureaucratic medicine,[49] research findings are translated into algorithmic clinical guidelines intended to operate as a kind of bureaucratic rule that governs the treatment of an entire category of patients. This approach is so naturalised within the UK healthcare system that the focus of research in this area is increasingly upon 'removing barriers' to the implementation of guidelines[50] rather than assessing whether or not the approach is likely to improve care in its widest sense. Within general practice, the increase in bureaucratic control exemplified by the new contract is justified for some by its potential to improve 'quality' and 'save lives'.[51] It is perhaps this conflation of the notion of 'quality' with the meeting of narrow biomedical targets,[52] which is the most worrying aspect of the evidence that we have presented here.

ACKNOWLEDGEMENTS

The English study was funded by the National Primary Care Research and Development Centre. The Scottish study was funded by the Economic and Social Research Council (ESRC) Public Services Programme and the East of Scotland Primary Care Research Network. We gratefully acknowledge the work of our coresearchers: Prof Ruth McDonald, Dr Suzanne Grant, Prof Bruce Guthrie and Dr Guro Huby. We are also indebted to the practices who took part, welcomed us into their practices and gave us their valuable time.

REFERENCES

1. Timmins N. Do GPs deserve their recent pay rise? *BMJ.* 2005; **331**(7520): 800.
2. Doran T, Fullwood C, Gravelle H, *et al.* Pay-for-performance programs in family practices in the United Kingdom. *N Engl J Med.* 2006; **355**(4): 375–84.
3. Checkland K, Harrison S, McDonald R, *et al.* Biomedicine, holism and general medical practice: responses to the 2004 General Practitioner contract. *Sociol Health Illn.* 2008; **30**(5): 788–803.

4. Murphy E, Dingwall R, Greatbatch D, *et al.* Qualitative research methods in health technology assessment: a review of the literature. *Health Technol Assess.* 1998; **2**(16): 1–275.

5. Checkland, Harrison, McDonald, *et al.*, op. cit.

6. Grant S, Huby G, Watkins F, *et al.* The impact of pay-for-performance on professional boundaries in UK general practice: an ethnographic study. *Sociol Health Illn.* 2009; **31**(2): 229–54.

7. Huby G, Guthrie B, Grant S, *et al.* Whither British General Practice after the 2004 GMS contract?: stories and realities of change in 4 UK general practices. *J Health Organ Manag.* 2008; **22**(1): 63–79.

8. Checkland K, McDonald R, Harrison S. Ticking boxes and changing the social world: data collection and the new UK general practice contract. *Soc Policy Adm.* 2007; **41**(7): 693–710.

9. McDonald R, Checkland K, Harrison S, *et al.* Rethinking collegiality: restratification in English general medical practice 2004–2008. *Soc Sci Med.* 2009; **68**(7): 1199–205.

10. McDonald R, Harrison S, Checkland K. Identity, contract and enterprise in a primary care setting: an English general practice case study. *Organization.* 2008; **15**(3): 355–70.

11. McDonald R, Harrison S, Checkland K, *et al.* Impact of financial incentives on clinical autonomy and internal motivation in primary care: ethnographic study. *BMJ.* 2007; **334**: 1357–9.

12. Royal College of General Practitioners. *Profile of UK Practices, August 2005. Information sheet no. 2.* London: RCGP; 2005.

13. Laing A, Marnoch G, McKee L, *et al.* Administration to innovation: the evolving management challenge in primary care. *J Manag Med.* 1997; **11**(2–3): 71–87.

14. Checkland K. Management in general practice: the challenge of the new General Medical Services contract. *Br J Gen Pract.* 2004; **54**(507): 734–9.

15. Checkland K. Understanding general practice: a conceptual framework from case studies in the UK National Health Service. *Br J Gen Pract.* 2007; **57**(534): 56–63.

16. NHS Executive. *Information for Health: an information strategy for the modern NHS 1998–2005.* London: The Stationary Office; 1998.

17. Elwyn G. Safety from numbers: identifying drug related morbidity using electronic records in primary care. *Qual Saf Health Care.* 2004; **13**(3): 170–1.

18. Hippisley-Cox J, Pringle M, Cater R, *et al.* The electronic patient record in primary care – regression or progression? A cross sectional study. *BMJ.* 2003; **326**(7404): 1439–43.

19. Laurence CO, Burgess T, Beilby J, *et al.* Electronic medical records may be inadequate for improving population health status through general practice: cervical smears as a case study. *Aust NZ J Public Health.* 2004; **28**(4): 317–20.

20. Williams PH, de Lusignan S. Does a higher 'quality points' score mean better care in stroke? An audit of general practice medical records. *Inform Prim Care.* 2006; **14**: 29–40.

21. Berg M. Practices of reading and writing: the constitutive role of the patient record in medical work. *Sociol Health Illn.* 1996; **18**(4): 499–524.

22. Berg M, Bowker G. The multiple bodies of the medical record: toward a sociology of an artifact. *Sociol Q.* 1997; **38**(3): 513–37.

23. Pinder R, Petchey R, Shaw S, *et al*. What's in a care pathway? Towards a cultural cartography of the new NHS. *Sociol Health Illn*. 2005; **27**(6): 759–79.
24. Cowley S, Mitcheson J, Houston AM. Structuring health needs assessments: the medicalisation of health visiting. *Sociol Health Illn*. 2004; **26**(5): 503–26.
25. Huby, Guthrie, Grant S, *et al.*, op. cit.
26. Jewson ND. The disappearance of the sick-man from medical cosmology, 1770–1870. *Sociology*. 1976; **10**(2): 225–44.
27. Cantor D. The diseased body. In: Cooter R, Pickstone JE, editors. *Medicine in the 20th Century*. London: Harwood; 2000. pp. 347–66.
28. Horder J, Byrne P, Freeling P, *et al*. *The Future General Practitioner: learning and teaching*. London: Royal College of General Practitioners; 1972.
29. Howie JGR, Heaney D, Maxwell M. Quality, core values and the general practice consultation: issues of definition, measurement and delivery. *Fam Pract*. 2004; **21**(4): 458–68.
30. Hasegawa H, Reilly D, Mercer SW, *et al*. Holism in primary care: the views of Scotland's general practitioners. *Prim Health Care Res Dev*. 2005; **6**(4): 320–9.
31. Mead N, Bower P. Patient-centred consultations and outcomes in primary care: a review of the literature. *Patient Educ Couns*. 2002; **48**(1): 51–61.
32. Sackett DL, Rosenberg WMC, Gray JAM, *et al*. Evidence based medicine: what it is and what it isn't. *Br Med J*. 1996; **312**(7023): 71–2.
33. Harrison S. New labour, modernisation and the medical labour process. *J Soc Policy*. 2002; **31**(3): 465–85.
34. Department of Health. *Delivering investment in General Practice: implementing the new GMS contract*. London: Department of Health; 2003.
35. NHS Confederation. *Briefing no 8: practice management under the new GMS contract*. London: NHS Confederation; 2003.
36. Checkland, Harrison, McDonald, *et al.*, op. cit.
37. Lervy B, Wareham K, Cheung WY. Practice characteristics associated with audit activity: a medical audit advisory group survey. *Br J Gen Pract*. 1994; **44**(384): 311–14.
38. Freidson E. The reorganisation of the medical profession. *Med Care Rev*. 1985; **42**(1): 11–35.
39. McDonald, Checkland, Harrison, *et al.*, op. cit.
40. Huby, Guthrie, Grant, *et al.*, op. cit.
41. Boyce ME. Organizational story and storytelling: a critical review. *J Organ Change Manag*. 1996; **9**(5): 5–26.
42. Harrison S. Co-optation, commodification and the medical model: governing UK medicine since 1991. *Public Adm*. 2009; **87**(2): 184–97.
43. Polanyi K. *The Great Transformation*. New York: Rinehart; 1944.
44. Esping-Andersen G. *The Three Worlds of Welfare Capitalism*. Cambridge: Polity Press; 1990.
45. Jeffries D. Save our soul. *Br J Gen Pract*. 2003; **53**(496): 888.
46. Harrison, op. cit.
47. Lawrence C. *Medicine and the Making of Modern Britain 1700–1920*. London: Routledge; 1994.
48. Pickstone JV. Ways of knowing: towards a historical sociology of science, technology and medicine. *Br J Hist Sci*. 1993; **26**: 433–58.
49. Harrison, op. cit.

50. Foy R, Walker A, Penney G. Barriers to clinical guidelines: the need for concerted action. *Br J Clin Govern.* 2001; **6**(3): 166–74.
51. Marshall M, Roland M. The new contract: renaissance or requiem for general practice? *Br J Gen Pract.* 2002; **52**(480): 531–2.
52. Loughlin M. 'Quality' and 'excellence': meaning versus rhetoric. In: Miles A, Hampton JR, Hurwitz B, editors. *NICE, CHI and the NHS Reforms: enabling excellence or imposing control?* London: Aesculapius Medical Press; 2000.

PART III

Practical aspects of the Quality and Outcomes Framework

CHAPTER 8

Getting the most out of the QOF

Chantal Simon and Anna Morton

SUMMARY

This chapter provides a practical approach to the Quality and Outcomes Framework (QOF) for general practitioners and practice teams. The QOF has brought a new dimension to target-driven pay in general practice, with practices currently paid around £124.60 per QOF point achieved, adjusted according to practice list size and characteristics. As the QOF payment forms a significant proportion of practice income, it is important for practices to achieve maximum points as efficiently as possible. This involves detailed knowledge of the QOF process, up-to-date awareness of QOF targets and the changes that are made to these year on year, forward planning and clear mechanisms within the practice to achieve these targets. As QOF points become increasingly difficult to attain, practices have to make difficult decisions about whether the time and effort required to achieve targets are worth the income derived.

Key points

- The QOF provides payment to practices for achievement of targets across both clinical and organisational domains.
- Knowledge of the QOF, forward planning and good organisation are essential to achieve a practice's maximum QOF potential.
- As targets become progressively harder to achieve, practices must make decisions about which targets to pursue.

INTRODUCTION

Introduction of the Quality and Outcomes Framework (QOF) has brought a new dimension to target-driven pay in general practice. The QOF is a voluntary process for all practices in the United Kingdom and awards practices points for managing common chronic diseases, e.g., asthma and diabetes; how well the practice is organised; how patients view their experience at the surgery; and extra services offered such as child health and maternity services.

In 2005/06, a year after the QOF was introduced, the average number of QOF points achieved by practices in England was 1010.5, representing 96.2% of the total 1050 points then available to each practice. Achievement in the clinical domains was even higher with the average practice earning 97.1% of the maximum 550 points available.

The QOF was designed to improve patient health and access to care. The number of practices receiving maximum points was much higher than originally anticipated. As a result, QOF standards were criticised for being set too low, and general practitioners (GPs) have been widely condemned for increasing their incomes without providing any improvement in services or care. With each QOF point being worth over £1 million across the United Kingdom, the 'QOF bonanza' was blamed for much overspending on primary care. This led to more demanding targets being set and that trend is likely to continue.

The average value of a QOF point was £124.60 in 2005/06 and has remained at that value ever since. More demanding targets have meant that practices have struggled to maintain their QOF achievement and the number of practices achieving maximum points dropped sharply between 2007/08 and 2008/09 (*see* Figure 8.1). This has resulted in QOF payments remaining relatively static compared to total primary care spend and thus accounting for a smaller proportion of total primary care spend than in previous years (*see* Figure 8.2).

The QOF income forms a substantial proportion of practice remuneration for most practices. However, getting systems in place to achieve as many QOF points as possible in 1 year will not ensure that the same income is derived in subsequent years. Each year, new targets are introduced and existing targets are changed, often making QOF points harder to obtain. As a result, practices are increasingly 'playing the QOF game'. Each year, they await publication of the year's new targets. Then,

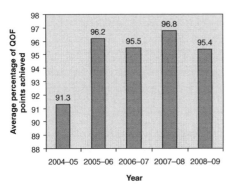
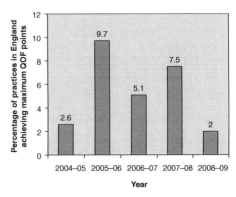

FIGURE 8.1 QOF achievement for English practices 2004/09. *Source:* NHS Information Centre for Health and Social Care

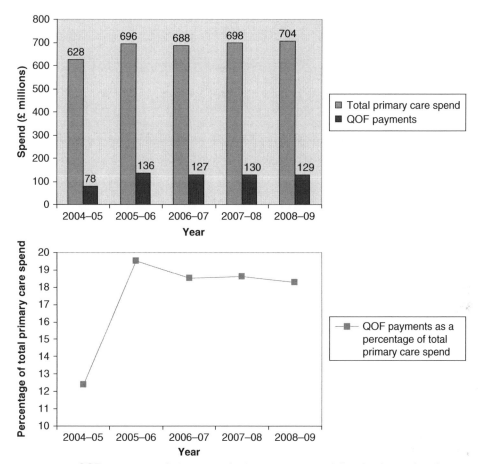

FIGURE 8.2 QOF payments relative to total primary care spend, Scotland 2004/09. *Source:* Investment in General Practice 2003/04 to 2008/09, England, Wales, Northern Ireland and Scotland (2009)

they devise ways to achieve maximum points with minimum work and financial expenditure. This chapter aims to define the rules of the 'QOF game' and explore some of the ways that practices currently use these rules to improve patient care while maintaining practice income.

QUALITY POINTS

For the QOF, all achievement against quality indicators converts to points. Each point has a monetary value. The exact monetary value of each point depends on practice characteristics and weighting for factors that increase work load through the allocation formula devised by Carr-Hill *et al.*[1] There are three main types of indicators, which are discussed in the following sections.

Yes/no indicators

All points are allocated if the result is positive, and none if it is negative. For example, records indicator 13 (Record 13) requires practices to have a system to alert the out-of-hours service or duty doctor to patients dying at home. The practice must be able to demonstrate the arrangements if required.[2,3]

Range of attainment

For most of the clinical indicators, it is not possible to attain 100% performance, even if allowed exceptions are applied, so a range of satisfactory attainment is specified. The minimum standard to gain any points is currently 40% for most indicators scored in this way. Points are allocated in a linear fashion based on comparison with attainment against a standard. For example, coronary heart disease indicator 7 (CHD 7) asks practices to report the percentage of their patients with CHD whose notes have a record of total cholesterol in the previous 15 months. Seven points are available with payment stages of 40–90%. If 65% of the practice patients do have a record of total cholesterol within the previous 15 months, then the practice will receive 25/50 (i.e., half) of the available points.[4]

Minimum standard indicators

All points are awarded if the criterion is met in more than a certain percentage of cases. For example, medicines indicator 12 (Medicine 12), worth 8 points, requires that a medication review is recorded in the notes in the preceding 15 months for at least 80% of patients being prescribed repeat medication.

EXCEPTION REPORTING

The QOF includes the concept of 'exception reporting'. This was introduced so that practices were not penalised where, e.g., patients do not attend for review, or where a medication cannot be prescribed due to a contraindication or side effect. Patient exception reporting applies to those indicators in the clinical domain of the QOF, where level of achievement is determined by the percentage of patients receiving the designated level of care. Exception reporting also applies to one of the cervical screening indicators in the additional services domain.

Valid exceptions are the following:

- Patients who have been recorded as refusing to attend review after being invited on at least three occasions during the preceding 12 months.
- Patients for whom it is not appropriate to review chronic disease parameters due to particular circumstances (e.g., those with terminal illness or extreme frailty) should be removed from the disease register for that condition, so that they do not affect the proportion of patients achieving targets.

- Patients newly diagnosed within the practice or who have recently registered with the practice should have measurements made within 3 months of registering and delivery of clinical standards within 9 months, e.g., achieving blood pressure or cholesterol measurements within target levels.
- Patients who are on maximum-tolerated doses of medication whose disease control remains suboptimal.
- Patients for whom prescribing a medication is not clinically appropriate, including those who have an allergy, another contraindication or who have experienced an adverse reaction to specific medications.
- Where a patient has not tolerated medication.
- Where a patient does not agree to investigation or treatment (informed dissent), and this has been recorded in the patient's medical records.
- Where the patient has a supervening condition that makes treatment of another medical condition inappropriate, e.g., cholesterol reduction where the patient has liver disease.
- Where an investigative or secondary care service is unavailable.

Practices should report the number of exceptions for each indicator set and individual indicator. Practices may be called to justify why they have 'excepted' patients from the QOF and the reasons for this should be identifiable in the clinical record.

For example, in a practice with 100 patients on the diabetes register, 86 (or 86%) have a record of presence or absence of peripheral pulses in the previous 15 months (DM 9) and the practice has not reached the 90% target required to receive the maximum points available. However, four patients have been recalled for follow-up to the in-house practice diabetic clinic on three occasions but have not attended. One patient has become terminally ill with metastatic breast carcinoma during the year, so it is inappropriate for her to attend further diabetic reviews. Therefore, only 95 patients could be checked and the practice has checked 86 of those patients (i.e., 86/95 or 91%) and is thus eligible for maximum points and maximum payment for that indicator.[5]

REPORTING ON QUALITY

Every year, each practice must complete a standard report recording level of achievement in the past year and the evidence for that. Most computerised practices use the quality management and analysis system (QMAS) system to do this (*see* later). In addition, there is an annual quality review visit by the practice's primary care organisation. The information provided by the practice is scrutinised and further evidence to back up the practice's data may be sought, e.g., through randomly checking records or asking practice staff about practice policies.[6,7,8]

The practice's points are totalled on 2nd April each year (National Achievement Day). The point value is adjusted according to factors in the Carr-Hill allocation formula, and also for prevalence of disease. For example, in a practice of 1000 patients catering for a university population, there are just four patients with a diagnosis of chronic obstructive pulmonary disease (COPD). This is because the practice population is young and the prevalence of COPD in this age group is low. Therefore, achieving high levels of attainment on the COPD indicators entails relatively little work.

As prevalence may vary through the year, prevalence is calculated in every practice across the United Kingdom every year on 14th February (14th March in Wales) ('National prevalence day'). Differences in prevalence data between practices expected to have similar populations may also be used to highlight practices that could be manipulating the QOF return and that require further investigation.

THE QOF MANAGEMENT AND ANALYSIS SYSTEM

The QMAS is software that has been developed for the new General Medical Services contract so that practices in England can assess their achievement under the new contract and contribute to the calculation of national disease prevalences.[9] Similar software is available in Scotland, Wales and Northern Ireland.

The central system collects the clinical and non-clinical achievement data, calculates the points/pounds and prevalences and displays the results. QMAS runs automatically for the QOF clinical indicators and a subset of the organisational and additional services indicators. Data relating to most of the organisational indicators cannot be automatically extracted and all practices need to enter organisation data manually. The QMAS system automatically calculates practice achievement and generates the final report.

PRACTICE STRUCTURE AND THE QOF

Although the trend for chronic disease management clinics started earlier, the advent of the QOF has changed practice staffing structure and working practices. The bulk of the clinical points within the QOF are available for chronic disease management, and most of the work to achieve these points is performed by practice nurses, using disease registers and call–recall systems. They work with protocols and disease-specific chronic disease management templates, in practice-based chronic disease management clinics.

Although this is an efficient way of completing as high a proportion of checks as possible, there are problems associated with this model of care. Especially, in larger practices where a single nurse often specialises in a single disease area, practices nurses and GPs can become deskilled. For example, it is not uncommon for a single patient with several chronic medical problems to be invited to three or four separate clinics because the nurses running these clinics are not skilled to perform all the disease checks required in a single appointment. Chronic disease management checks are repetitive and can result in job dissatisfaction.

Although practice nurses are doing the bulk of the work to achieve clinical targets, the considerable sums generated through the QOF go into the practice 'pot'. Practice nurses usually receive much lower pay than the GPs running the practice, yet any extra profit achieved from reaching QOF targets is divided between the partners running the practice. It is easy for resentment to grow and therefore important for those doing the work to feel appreciated. Financial incentives built into employment contracts may help. The QOF has also increased the number of administrative staff within most practices. Even quite small practices may employ someone simply to ensure the smooth running of the QOF.

Finally, the QOF has dramatically increased practice workload. A great deal of administrative and investigative work is required for GPs. Regular checks flag up disease-related problems that GPs are asked to deal with. Regular contact and familiarity with practice nurses in chronic disease management clinics also gives patients opportunities to bring up other medical problems about which they might not usually have consulted. In most cases, the nurses running the chronic disease management clinics cannot deal with such queries. This, in turn, generates a need for further GP appointments.

GETTING THE MOST OUT OF THE QOF

Box 8.1 summarises the ways that practices can maximise their chances of getting QOF points.

Box 8.1 Top 10 tips for obtaining QOF points
1   Know the rules
2   Plan your strategy at the start of the year
3   Work at your QOF targets all year
4   Involve the whole team effectively
5   Use your practice computer system efficiently
6   Actively target specific patient groups
7   Maximise points for patients on multiple disease registers
8   Scrutinise exception reporting
9   Think laterally
10 Link QOF to other practice activities, e.g., practice-based commissioning or prescribing targets

---

Know the rules

The QOF is complex, is also under continual review and updates at intervals. It is important to know what is required for each standard. Invest in training where necessary (*see* Box 8.2).

Box 8.2 Understanding the QOF rules

The Willow practice has produced an interim report on how they are getting on with new depression targets in the revised QOF. They think that they all have been recording depression correctly. They get a nasty shock, on finding that they are a long way off their targets for depression indicator 3 (DEP 3), worth up to 20 points:

In those patients with a new diagnosis of depression and assessment of severity recorded between the preceding 1 April to 31 March, the percentage of patients who have had a further assessment of severity, 5–12 weeks (inclusive) after the initial recording of the assessment of severity. Both assessments should be completed using an assessment tool validated for use in primary care.

Dr Patel has been asked to look at the data and work out what they are doing wrong. When this indicator was first announced, a new system of managing patients with depression was introduced into the practice. It was agreed that on first presentation, clinicians would assess severity of depression by completing a Patient Health Questionnaire (PHQ-9) with the patient and recording the result on computer. The hard copy of the questionnaire would then be scanned onto the computer. Follow-up would routinely take place 2 weeks after initial diagnosis and then again a few months later. At this second follow-up, a repeat PHQ-9 questionnaire would be completed.

On review of the patient records, Dr Patel noted that clinicians did seem to be reviewing patients and using the assessment tools as directed. However, at follow-up, several GPs were giving the patient the depression questionnaire to self-complete. The patients were being asked to hand the completed questionnaire to the receptionist. A questionnaire recording severity of depression at follow-up had been scanned onto the computer, but there was no READ-coded 'score' of severity of depression recorded at this time, making it appear as if the assessments had not been done.

The codes for the follow-up assessments that had been done but not correctly recorded were added. This brought the total percentage up to 80%, which was better but still not up to the 90% required for maximum points.

While going through the notes, Dr Patel also found several patients with recurrences of depression who had been recorded as having new depression. DEP3 applies to patients with a new diagnosis of depression only. Examination of the records of the 20% who had not had an assessment with a validated tool 5–12 weeks after initial recording of severity showed that nearly half had a previous diagnosis of depression. He recoded the diagnosis to 'recurrent depression' for these individuals and the practice exceeded the 90% for maximum QOF points.

Plan your strategy at the start of the year

Planning is essential to maximise QOF income. It is too late to do much about unmet targets if failure to achieve the required standards is flagged too late in the year. Before the start of the financial year, meet to:

- look at the changes to the QOF from the previous year, such as new standards, changes in targets required or changes in the rules; work out how these can be incorporated into the existing systems that you already have in place
- look at ways in which the system used the previous year can be improved
- identify areas of the QOF that the practice performs well in, and areas where there could be improvement; do not forget the non-clinical areas
- target the processes and QOF domains identified for improvement and assign each QOF area to a member of the clinical or administration team; this ensures a named individual becomes a specialist in the requirements for that area and is responsible for monitoring progress

Work at your QOF targets all year

Ensure regular internal interim QOF reviews. If the practice is falling behind on one standard, then have a drive to increase achievement levels. In addition to recording for clinical targets, make a record of evidence supporting organisational markers in order to facilitate future primary care organisation (PCO) visits (*see* Box 8.3).

Involve the whole team efficiently

The income generated by the QOF affects the whole practice. All staff, including receptionists and administration staff, should be aware of this and take responsibility for achieving the maximum QOF points available. If staff are not getting involved with maximising QOF achievement, is it because they do not understand its importance, in health and financial terms? Alternatively, is it because they feel they do not have time or it is not their job?

Make sure that everyone knows what they should be doing. Consider staff training sessions, reviewing job descriptions and changing induction procedures to ensure staff understand why maximising QOF achievement is important and what their roles are. Include staff actions that affect QOF income in contracts of

Box 8.3 Developing systems for achieving the QOF targets

It was noticed 3 months into the year that none of the patients registered with Stopples practice who were recorded as having dementia had a care review recorded in their notes, even though several had been seen for other reasons, such as minor infections. Although the number of patients was relatively small, there were 15 potential QOF points at stake. Dr May was asked to do something about it.

She downloaded a list of the 66 patients with a diagnosis of dementia registered with the practice. Of these, 16 were permanent residents in care homes within the practice area. One care home registered to take residents with dementia was home to 10 of these patients. She rang the care home and arranged a time to go there and review all these patients in one go. She also put a prominent note above the visit book asking any other GP visiting care homes, where the other patients with dementia were resident to do their reviews opportunistically while visiting.

Of the remaining 50 patients, 25 were under regular follow-up in the practice for other reasons, such as hypertension or diabetes monitoring. The practice nurses running these clinics were reminded of the need to undertake dementia reviews for these patients using the template on the practice computer when they came for their routine checks. A flag was placed on the computer notes of patients concerned to alert the practice nurses to do this.

A further 15 patients were seen from time to time by the district nurses in the community. A discussion with Jenny, the district nurse attached to the practice, revealed that she had recently undertaken dementia reviews for 11 of these patients as part of her routine assessment. These were recorded in her notes but not on the practice computer. Her reviews were added to the practice computer.

All those patients not seeing the district nurse, not a resident in a care home and not attending the practice for regular reviews for other reasons were contacted by letter. They and/or their carers were invited either to make an appointment, to come to the practice, or to ring for a GP to visit for routine review. In addition, the GPs and nurse practitioner were reminded that these reviews could be done opportunistically if they saw the patient for any other reason. Flags were placed on the patients' notes to alert clinicians that a dementia review was required.

Less than a month after identifying the problem, more than 60% of the patients had a dementia review recorded ensuring that all 15 QOF points could be claimed.

employment (e.g., the need to attend training in basic life support skills at regular intervals). Consider performance-related pay or bonuses for key staff such as the practice manager for delivering improved QOF achievement.

Use your practice computer effectively

All licensed general practice software now includes mechanisms to record QOF data. Since searches are done on specific READ codes, it is important to ensure that the correct READ codes are entered to enable the computer to extract all relevant information. Every system does this slightly differently, so it is important to ensure

---

Box 8.4 Involving the team

The Copse Surgery noticed as the year end approaches that the percentage of patients aged over 15 years whose notes record 'never smoked' or smoking status in the past 27 months was only 76%. Dr Green was dispatched to deal with the problem.

He asked the computer manager to add a prompt to flash up on screen whenever any patient's notes without a smoking status record, or with a record added more than a year previously of the patient being a smoker or ex-smoker, were accessed. He asked all of those in direct patient contact (doctors, nurses and reception staff) to ask patients their smoking status if they spotted the prompt box and put a large notice up in each consulting room to remind clinical staff. He also asked the repeat prescribing clerk to attach a letter to repeat prescriptions, asking patients without a recent smoking status or never smoked record to let the practice know whether and how much they smoke.

Two weeks later, he reviewed the situation. Although the percentage had gone up to 79%, there was still some way to reach the 90% target. Checking a random sample of patients without a recent record, he noted that most were not regular attenders at the surgery. It was therefore difficult to target them via direct encounters. He proposed two evening telephone sessions when receptionists were paid to come in to ring all those on the list of patients with no recent record of smoking status. The proposal was approved. After four frantic hours of telephoning, the percentage was up to 90.8%.

Afterwards, there was a meeting to discuss what went wrong. Several factors emerged. Many of the patients recorded as ex-smokers on the computer had only tried one or two cigarettes ever. It was agreed that these patients should be recoded as non-smokers and then, once over the age of 25, will not need to be asked their smoking status every 27 months. Everyone also agreed that next year's smoking data should be collected throughout the year, especially for new registrations and when infrequent attenders come to the surgery.

that everyone entering data is aware of how to do it and which terms they should be using on your system.

Many software systems include review programmes or disease templates. The clinician (or another staff member) can work through the programme for any given QOF domain (e.g., heart failure) and the programme will automatically prompt the clinician to enter the information required and code it using the correct READ codes.

Another feature on many systems is a summary of each QOF domain. This can be accessed via the patient's notes to establish whether the patient should be included on the disease register and what other information is needed. Often this information can be entered directly through the QOF summary screen into the patient's notes and again the correct READ codes are automatically supplied.

At a local level, recording patient data can be made easier by altering the default terms. For example, most people coming to the surgery about atrial fibrillation (AF) will already have it. When 'AF' is typed into the computer, it is more sensible to default to 'AF review' than 'atrial fibrillation', which is identified in the QOF as a new diagnosis of AF and therefore requires confirmation of diagnosis with electro-cardiogram or by a specialist.

Most systems also enable practices to insert prompts for anyone using the system. For example, a box may flash up when that patient's notes are accessed reminding users that the patient is on specific disease registers, has an overdue smear, needs a coil check, etc. This can be an effective way to remind clinicians to collect data needed or to do other tasks for QOF purposes. However, if prompt boxes appear on every screen, it is easier for staff to ignore them. Ensure that any prompts are correct and conform to current policies.

Make good use of other information technology tools including an add-on management and planning tool such as 'contract manager'. It is recommended that practices make an extra backup shortly after 1st April each year and keep this for 7 years in case there is any need to verify claims made under the QOF.

Actively target specific patient groups

Targeting specific patient groups is important to achieve maximum QOF points for several reasons. Annual patient reviews conducted between January and March each year may count towards 2 years' points calculation as the criteria often look back 15 months from the financial year-end reference date.

Patients with chronic diseases earning QOF points generate a lot of money for a practice. Make sure that your disease registers are accurate. Wrongly diagnosed and thus untreated patients will count against your percentage achievement. It is also important to ensure that regular reviews take place and all data required are recorded at each review using templates and reminders to ensure that nothing is missed. Most practices use nurse-led clinics to follow-up their patients with the chronic diseases that generate the most points, such as diabetes mellitus, hypertension, asthma, COPD, stroke and CHD.

Smokers can potentially earn a large number of QOF points for a practice (81 currently). Points are available for recording whether a patient is a smoker and providing smoking cessation advice and information.

Infrequent attenders can be a problem for practices collecting QOF data. Some QOF targets require information from all patients, even those without medical problems. Examples include blood pressure data every 5 years for all those aged over 45, and smoking data for all those aged 15 or over. These data should be collected opportunistically whenever these patients come to the surgery. It is hard to access these patients otherwise.

Look at prevalence

If disease prevalence is lower than the average, the practice will lose points through prevalence adjustments, so it is important to ensure that patients with chronic diseases are included on disease registers. If prevalence is still low, target high-risk groups to ensure that patients with these chronic diseases are not being missed. This is also important as QOF assessors may challenge the practice return if prevalence is not as expected. It is important to be able to justify your figures.

Maximise points for patients on multiple disease registers

Many patients have multiple chronic diseases. For example, it is not uncommon for a single individual to be obese, smoker, have CHD, COPD, chronic kidney disease, diabetes mellitus and a history of stroke. That patient is very valuable to the practice, as he or she can potentially contribute to more than 250 QOF points for the practice. It is important to make sure that reviews for these multiple category patients take place, as missing reviews can affect multiple targets. There are many common elements in the reviews required for several of the domains, so combining routine reviews for all the conditions affecting that patient is both a cost- and time-effective way of maximising QOF points. Measure and record all relevant information about a patient in one visit using templates and reminders to make sure that you do not miss anything.

Scrutinise exception reporting

The overall exception rate for England, across all indicator groups, is just over 5% (*see* Chapter 6). There is a considerable variation in exception rates across the indicators. In general, the lowest exception rates are observed in relation to indicators that measure a process, such as recording smoking or blood pressure. The highest exception rates are observed in relation to indicators that measure outcome, such as HbA1c level.

Look at your practice exception rate compared with national and local figures. If you are excepting too many patients, check that you can justify your exceptions. If you are excepting too few patients, look at your disease registers and the exception criteria. Is there anyone else on the disease register who should be excepted?

Box 8.5 Exception reporting

Jane, the nurse running the cardiovascular clinic in the Beech Practice, had a big push to review patients with heart failure. She was disappointed when told that she had fallen just short of the maximum points target for the percentage on an angiotensin-converting enzyme inhibitor (ACEI) or angiotensin receptor blocker (ARB).

There were 144 patients registered with the practice with heart failure—112 of them were on an ACEI/ARB (78%). She printed off a list of patients on the heart failure register but not on an ACEI or ARB, and started checking their notes. Five patients had terminal illnesses (two widespread metastatic cancer, one end-stage dementia, one advanced Parkinson's disease and one motor neurone disease). They were valid exceptions. This took the denominator down to 139, and the percentage on an ACEI/ARB to 81% qualifying for maximum payment.

Think laterally

Every practice is different but there are many ways in which individual practices have made data collection for QOF purposes easier. The following are real examples from practices we have experience of:

- Give every patient a brief questionnaire asking height, weight, smoking status and alcohol consumption to complete in the waiting room while waiting for any appointment to return to the receptionist.
- Consider installing a self-service blood pressure monitor allowing patients to check their own blood pressure in the waiting room. Ensure blood pressures checked in this way are automatically recorded on computer or given to the receptionist before the patient leaves.
- At the time of the annual influenza vaccination clinics, consider trawling patients expected to attend for those who have defaulted from chronic disease management clinics. Ensure a clinician is present at each 'flu clinic' who can target and perform basic QOF checks on these patients while they are in the surgery.
- Remember to record ethnicity when registering newborn babies.

Link to other practice activities

The QOF is only one element in the running of a practice. QOF activities should not be seen in isolation. Try to link QOF activity into other practice activities to economise on resources. For example, link reviews of medication to prescribing reviews. Consider QOF needs when thinking about priorities for practice-based commissioning.

DECIDING ENOUGH IS ENOUGH

With increasing financial pressures on practices, and more competition from other providers, the temptation is to try to achieve every QOF point. However, as QOF points become harder to achieve, when does chasing every QOF point cease to be cost-effective?

When deciding whether to attempt to attain a new QOF target, it is important to weigh-up the pros and cons. First, it is important to find out precisely what achieving the target will entail.

Most new QOF targets require the practice to undertake additional work. How much work will be needed in this instance? For example, do we already record the relevant data (in which case, it will be relatively simple to extract) or will we have to start recording the data from scratch?

If additional work is needed, it is important to look at who will do that work and how much that additional work will cost the practice. If the additional work is simply an extra question to ask during a routine diabetic check, then the practice nurse running the clinic should be able to do it without any extra cost to the practice. If the additional work involves extending staff hours, or even employing a new member of staff, then this may entail considerable expense to the practice.

If meeting a new target entails extra expense, it is important to weigh-up whether that additional expenditure is counterbalanced either by the additional income or other benefits to the practice, e.g., in terms of better patient care. As targets become more difficult to achieve, practices have to make difficult decisions. For each new target, the practice needs to decide whether achieving that target is in the interests of their patients, GPs and other staff. If the answer to that question is 'no', then the next question has to be: can we afford *not* to provide this service?

Box 8.6 Weighing the benefits

Note: This example involves a fictional change to the QOF!

The team at the Galaxy practice were reviewing changes to the following year's QOF. They noticed a major change in the obesity domain. Up until now, the practice has simply been required to keep a register of patients aged 16 and over with a body mass index (BMI) over 30 recorded in the previous 15 months. There was no requirement to measure the BMI of every patient.

This year, a new target requires the practice to measure BMI once every 5 years for everyone over the age of 16 on the practice list. The target is worth 4 points with a range of achievement from 40 to 90%. Each point is worth £124.60, so it was estimated that achieving the target would bring the practice £498.40 in a year.

There were 4044 patients over the age of 16 on the practice list; 33% had had their BMI recorded in the past 5 years. Eight per cent attend the practice on a regular basis for contraceptive checks. Forty-two per cent attend for chronic disease management checks of some sort. A further 6% attend for new patient checks or well man/woman checks. Therefore, 56% could have their BMI recorded relatively easily.

However, just over 14% of the practice population had not been seen at all in the surgery in the past 5 years. Even if everyone coming to the surgery to see the GP was weighed, the maximum percentage that could have been achieved was 86%. Accessing this hidden 14% would be difficult, requiring much work from the practice for little gain. This outlay was not thought to be justified.

The practice could easily achieve the lower payment target, so it was decided that patients not attending the practice for routine checks would be weighed opportunistically. In addition, a weighing machine was placed in reception to allow patients to weigh themselves and record their weight directly onto the practice computer. In this way, patients who did not routinely attend for themselves (e.g., working men attending with wives or children, or carers) might also be seen.

By the following year, 80% of patients had been weighed and the practice achieved four fifths of the money available (£398.72), with an outlay of £350 for the electronic scales in reception. Therefore, a profit of £48.72 was made. The following year, the figure was 82% with a £45 outlay for servicing of the scales, giving a much healthier profit of £363.69.

CONCLUSIONS

The QOF has become a powerful force influencing every aspect of primary care practice in the United Kingdom. Although designed to improve patient care, QOF achievement is largely decided on the basis of the quality of data collected by a practice. This results in both clinical and administrative challenges for practices. Furthermore, the QOF is not static, but constantly changing and thereby placing ever more demands on practices. It is essential for practices to stay on top of QOF developments, plan ahead and involve the whole practice team if they are to achieve their maximum QOF potential.

ACKNOWLEDGEMENTS

We thank Mrs Iris Pilgrim, Practice Manager, Totton Health Centre, Southampton; Dr Maryanne Falle, GP QOF lead, Totton Health Centre, Southampton; and Mrs Ramona Boston-Strange, Cardiovascular Specialist Nurse, The Banks and Bearwood Medical Centres, Bournemouth, for their help with reviewing this chapter.

REFERENCES

1. Carr-Hill RA, Sheldon TA, Smith P, *et al.* Allocating resources to health authorities: development of method for small area analysis of use of inpatient services. *BMJ.* 1994; **309**: 1046–9.
2. Harvey J, Bateman C, Pittarides R, *et al. Handbook of Practice Management.* London: RSM Press; 2000 and updates.
3. Simon C. The Quality and Outcomes Framework. *InnovAiT.* 2008; **1**(3): 206–13.
4. NHS Employers. *Quality Outcomes Framework 2009/10.* Available at: www.nhsemployers. org/Aboutus/Publications/Documents/QOF_Guidance_2009_final.pdf
5. Department of Health. *Quality and Outcomes Framework.* Available at: www.dh.gov.uk/ en/Policyandguidance/Organisationpolicy/Primarycare/Primarycarecontracting/ QOF/index.htm
6. BMA. *Quality and Outcomes Framework.* Available at: www.bma.org.uk/ap.nsf/ Content/Hubqualityandoutcomes
7. NHS Information Centre for Health and Social Care. *Investment in General Practice 2003/4–2008/9 England, Wales, Northern Ireland and Scotland;* 2009. Available at: www. ic.nhs.uk/statistics-and-data-collections/primary-care/general-practice/investment-in-general-practice-2003-04-to-2007-08-england-wales-and-northern-ireland (accessed 8 July 2010).
8. NHS. *The Information Centre for Health and Social Care – QOF results 2008/9.* Available at: www.qof.ic.nhs.uk
9. NHS Connecting for Health. *What is QMAS?* Available at: www.connectingforhealth. nhs.uk/delivery/programmes/qmas
10. iSD Scotland. *Quality & Outcomes Framework (QOF) of the new General Medical Services Contract. Achievement, Exception Reporting and Detailed Prevalence Data 2008/09.* Available at: www.isdscotland.org/isd/6025.html

CHAPTER 9

Does the patient always benefit?

Patricia Wilkie

SUMMARY

The Quality and Outcomes Framework (QOF) was introduced to improve the quality of care for patients in general practice. Since its introduction, research has been carried out into improvements in clinical standards, public health and organisational changes, which may have resulted. However, such research is invariably from the medical or managerial perspective. Although some studies refer to possible effects of the QOF on patient care, there does not appear to be any substantive work from the lay perspective. In this chapter, some of the implications of the QOF are examined from a patient perspective.

Key points
- There has been little substantive research on the impact of the QOF from the lay or patient perspective.
- Aspects of patient care that are not subject to financial incentives may be given lower priority.
- The relationship between patient and general practitioner may be adversely affected by focusing on meeting targets rather than the patient's agenda.
- As nurses see most patients with chronic conditions, there is a risk that doctors will become deskilled in these clinical areas, previously seen as part of their job.
- Some patient-related aspects of care such as being able to book an appointment in advance or consult a practitioner of choice have not improved with introduction of the QOF.
- General practice work is becoming increasingly divided among salaried doctors, specialist nurses and other members of the practice team with the risk that no one is looking after the whole person.
- An explanation of why QOF data are being collected should be provided to patients.

BREAKING NEW GROUND

The philosophy behind the introduction of the Quality and Outcomes Framework (QOF) in 2004 was to raise national standards of primary care. The government wished to demonstrate to the public that they could expect a high standard of care from their general practice regardless of whom the patient was and where they lived. Both the government and the medical profession were aware that there were a number of general practitioners (GPs) offering suboptimal patient care.

Initially, the majority of practices were able to achieve the targets set and there was evidence of improvements in some clinical areas relating to chronic disease.[1,2] This undoubtedly has made a difference to individual patients. However, as described in earlier chapters, there is evidence that the quality of care for some chronic conditions had already been improving prior to the introduction of the QOF.

Rewarding GPs financially for achieving a broad range of targets has been a fairly new departure for UK general practice. However, it was introduced with apparently little research into both how such an incentive scheme might change the delivery of care by GPs, and its possible effect on the relationship between patients and their doctors. Although the QOF embraces a market model of healthcare with performance linked to bonuses (pay-for-performance),[3] the collection of QOF data involves considerable work and little spare capacity for other work in the majority of general practices. A possible consequence of the effort required to focus on the QOF is that attention to aspects of patient care that are not subject to financial incentives may be given lower priority and less time. They may even be marginalised to the possible detriment of some patients. Since the QOF only measures certain aspects of care, it is difficult to be sure that the quality of care in other area has not declined as QOF targets are prioritised or to know what harm may occur as a result of future activities, which are no longer prioritised in the QOF. Practice nurses, among others, have suggested that that the delivery of QOF targets has led to the detriment of overall patient care.[4]

CHANGING PROFESSIONAL PRACTICE

Mangin and Toop[5] argue that the central issue is not whether GPs should be paid for achieving targets nor whether the QOF indicators chosen are appropriate, but a philosophical concern with the nature of professionalism, professional values and the concept of good care.

What patients want from general practice is quality care given by a competent professional who is up to date, who knows the patient and who involves the patient in decision making.[6] Thus, the focus for both patients and professionals should be 'patient centredness' as a core value of general practice. With the emphasis in practices now on the collection of QOF data, there is a real danger that the needs of individual patients will not always be met. This could result in the relationship between the patient and their GP being adversely affected. For example, will the professional in the consultation always be focusing on the patient's agenda or are they distracted by the need to collect QOF data?

Campbell et al.,[7] in their qualitative study of doctors and nurses, found that the QOF was perceived as changing the agenda in the consultation for both doctors and nurses by encouraging them to focus on targets as well as addressing the concerns of the patient. Although doctors and nurses reported that they would give priority to the concerns of the patient, the authors suggest that addressing the QOF might make shared decision making difficult within the time constraints of a 10-minute consultation.

There is also anecdotal evidence from individual patients and some patient organisations that both GPs and practice nurses are focusing more on questions that seem irrelevant to the patient. A recent report from a slim, active 69-year-old patient attending for influenza vaccine illustrates the point. The patient was faced with questions about diet, smoking, exercise and alcohol consumption. There was no explanation for why these questions were asked; they seemed irrelevant to having a 'flu vaccine.' Blood pressure and weight had to be recorded and a cholesterol test organised. A short appointment lasted almost 15 minutes without the patient having the opportunity to ask a question about any aspect of 'flu vaccine. Although it is appreciated that staff need to take the opportunity of collecting data from patients who may not attend frequently, all healthcare professionals need to learn the skills required to ensure that collecting QOF data does not prevent the patient from asking questions nor impede joint decision making. In other words, activities for the QOF must be incorporated as part of patient-centred care.

Another aspect of concern to patients is the possible deskilling of practitioners. With the emphasis on evidence-based targets and with nurses seeing the majority of patients with chronic conditions, there is a danger that doctors could become deskilled in areas previously seen as part of their job. New recruits to general practice will not know anything else. Patients with a chronic condition such as asthma or diabetes do not want to be labelled as an asthmatic or diabetic. They live with the condition but may have other health problems quite unrelated to the chronic condition and need the generalist skills of a competent GP.

Patients value being cared for by a clinician who is a good diagnostician and who knows the patient and their circumstances; they also value continuity of care.[8] There is considerable evidence of the fragmentation in the management of care of long-term conditions such as diabetes in the secondary care sector.[9] In 1997, the journalist John Hoyland[10] described the hospital care of his octogenarian father-in-law treated by three different specialists for Parkinson's disease, arthritis and an enlarged prostrate, and shunted between three different hospitals. 'The problem was that while there were lots of people in charge of different parts of Jack's body, no one was in charge of Jack'.[11]

Traditionally, fragmentation of care has not been a problem in general practice where at the outset of the National Health Service (NHS), GPs alone provided continuity of care from the cradle to the grave. Most patients were looked after by a GP who knew the patient and their circumstances. General practice has now changed, with patients no longer being registered with an individual doctor (previously referred by patients as 'my doctor'), but instead with the practice now responsible for providing continuity of care. There is also evidence that patients have difficulties in seeing the doctor of their choice making it more difficult to maintain continuity.[12]

WHAT PATIENTS WANT?

The National Patient Survey has questions on specific aspects of continuity of care. These concern being able to consult the doctor of ones choice and being able to book an appointment in advance. Although the QOF does not have explicit questions about continuity, practices were required to undertake a patient survey using either the general practice assessment questionnaire (GPAQ) or the improving practice questionnaire (IPQ). Both these questionnaires have questions about access and seeing the doctor of one's choice. While Baker et al. did not demonstrate explicitly that the QOF had impaired continuity,[13] their study did show that the patient experience indicators within the QOF such as being able to book an appointment in advance or being able to consult a practitioner of choice have not improved. However, from a patient perspective, these are rather limited measurements of continuity. As continuity is so valued by patients and many GPs, it would be good to see this aspect strengthened in future developments of the QOF.

Another area that should be included in the QOF concerns the early recognition, diagnosis and management of the patient's presenting problem. Patients want help with their presenting medical problem and improvement for the patient is more likely when both the professional and the patient agree about this. As yet the early recognition of acute problems has not been incorporated into the QOF, but patients' experience might be improved were this to be the case.[14]

In recent years, more nurses are being employed in general practice with the numbers of consultations being carried out by nurses also increasing.[15] The 1990 GP Contract paid doctors to meet population targets for immunisation, vaccination and cervical cytology as well as to set up health prevention and health promotion clinics. Practices responded by employing nurses to carry out these roles. However, unlike the 1990 contract which was with individual GPs, the 2004 contract is with the practice, making it easier for practices to substitute nurses for doctors. Furthermore, there are indications that practices have increased the use of nurses working in extended roles including the collection of QOF data.[16] Sibbald[17] suggests that nurses can effectively deliver most clinical care in general practice leaving doctors to deal with that minority of patients who have complex medical problems. There is a danger that the QOF with its focus on diseases may result in care that omits to look at the whole person to the detriment of the patient. The work of the once expert 'generalist' GP is becoming increasingly divided among salaried doctors, specialist nurses and other members of the practice team[18,19,20] with the resulting danger that no one, just as for Jack, is looking after the whole person.

Angela Coulter from the Picker Institute has stated that a sustainable and responsive healthcare system should include transparency and public accountability for policy decisions,[21] a notion that is widely endorsed and incorporated in the seven Nolan principles for the conduct of public life.[22] Although the public still rate doctors highly in Ipsos MORI and other similar polls, there has been mounting public criticism of GP services around access, out-of-hours provision, lack of continuity of care and professional standards as reflected in some high-profile General Medical Council (GMC) disciplinary cases. The medical profession has also felt a lack of public trust and reduced status and this may have partly resulted in many articles about medical professionalism.[23] O'Neill[24] suggests that considerable effort has been made in the United Kingdom in recent years to develop trustworthiness by constructing a more open public culture, by abolishing traditions of secrecy and ensuring greater transparency. It is therefore disappointing that there has been a lack of comprehensible information for the public about the QOF; it is unlikely that the majority of patients know much about the QOF.

Patient involvement means not only involving patients in decisions about their individual care but also involving patients in the organisation of the NHS. From a patient's perspective, an explanation of why QOF data are being collected should be provided. Ideally, such information should be displayed in the waiting room or in practice leaflets and could be publicised by patient participation groups and patients' organisations such as National Association for Patient Participation. This would help patients understand why QOF-related questions are asked, and it might also be beneficial to practitioners. Informing patients about QOFs is a mature way of working with patients and could help to develop trust between the public and the health professionals.

As new QOF domains are introduced and the domains tightened, it has gradually become more difficult for some practices to attain the targets and thus the linked financial rewards. The link between QOF targets and financial rewards can raise doubts in the mind of patients. Connell,[25] writing of his experiences both as a doctor and a potential patient, could be described as an informed patient. He invites the question that some patients may ask: 'is this investigation for my own need or is to achieve a bonus?' He goes on to develop his own charter where care will be based on longstanding continuity and where he, the patient, knows that his doctor will have no conflict of interest: money will not get in the way of trust.

CONCLUSIONS

The introduction of the QOF has benefited some patients with chronic diseases by improving the management of these conditions. It is also hoped that the public health preventive measures included in the QOF will benefit many. However, for patients, there are real concerns about weakening continuity of care, which may be partly attributed to the QOF. There is also a danger that clinicians will find it increasingly difficult to offer patient-centred care. The GMC in 'Tomorrow's Doctors'[26] states that 'to justify trust doctors must make the care of the patient their first concern'. Most doctors wish to do this but it will take increasing skill to maintain the trust of patients, by balancing the demands of the QOF with the professional obligation to work in partnership with patients, so as to make care of the patient their first concern.

REFERENCES

1. Tahrani AA, McCarthy M, Gordon J, *et al.* Diabetes care and the new contract: the evidence for a whole country. *Br J Gen Pract.* 2007; **57**: 483–5.
2. Steel N, Maisey S, Clark A, *et al.* Quality of primary care and targeted incentive payments: an observational study. *Br J Gen Pract.* 2007; **57**: 449–54.
3. Mangin D, Toop L. The Quality and Outcomes Framework: what have you done to yourselves? *Br J Gen Pract.* 2007; **57**(539): 435–7.
4. *Health Care Republic QOF Nurse Survey – Are Targets Damaging Patient Care?* Available at: www.healthcarerepublic.com/news/772331/
5. Mangin, Toop, op. cit.
6. Coulter A, Elwyn G. What do patients want from high-quality general practice and how do we involve them in improvement? *Br J Gen Pract.* 2002; **52** (Suppl): S22–6.
7. Campbell SM, McDonald R, Lester H. The experience of pay for performance in English family practice: a qualitative study. *Ann Fam Med.* 2008; **6**: 228–34.
8. *Health Care Republic QOF Nurse Survey,* op. cit.
9. Gulliford MC, Naithani S, Morgan M. Measuring continuity of care in diabetes mellitus: an experience-based measure. *Ann Fam Med.* 2006; **4**: 548–55.
10. Wilkie P. The person, the patient and their carers. In: Faull C, Carter Y, Woof R, editors. *Handbook of Palliative Care.* Oxford: Blackwell; 1998. pp. 55–63.
11. Gulliford, Naithani, Morgan, op. cit.
12. *Health Care Republic QOF Nurse Survey,* op. cit.
13. Baker R, Bankart MJ, Murtagh GM. Do the quality and outcome framework patient experience indicators reward practices that offer improved access. *Br J Gen Pract.* 2009; **50**(565): 584–9.
14. Starfield B, Shi I, Macinko J. Contributions of primary care to health systems and health. *Millbank Q.* 2005; **83**: 457–50.
15. Sibbald B. Who needs doctors in general practice? *Qual Prim Care.* 2008; **16**: 73–4.
16. *Health Care Republic QOF Nurse Survey,* op. cit.
17. Sibbald, op. cit.
18. Hippisley-Cox J, Pringle M. General practice workload implications of the National Service Framework for coronary heart disease: cross sectional survey. *BMJ.* 2001; **323**: 269–70.
19. Barr R. Quality in practice. *Nurs Stand.* 2005; **19**: 22–3.
20. Griffiths P, Murrells T, Mahen J, *et al.* Nurse staffing and quality of care in UK general practice: cross-sectional study using routinely collected data. *Br J Gen Pract.* 2010; **60**: 34–9.

21. Picker Institute. *Annual Review 2005/6. Being treated like a person not a number, that's what counts for me.* Oxford: Picker Institute Europe; 2006.

22. Nolan Committee. *First Report of the Committee on Standards in Public Life.* London: HMSO; 1995.

23. Royal College of Physicians. *Doctors in Society; Medical Professionalism in a Changing Society.* London: RCP; 2005.

24. O'Neill O. *Autonomy and Trust in Bioethics.* Cambridge: Cambridge University Press; 2002.

25. Connell DG. Patient care – crunch time. *Br J Gen Pract.* 2009; 59: 546.

26. General Medical Council. *Tomorrow's Doctors.* London: General Medical Council; 2003.

PART IV

Reflections on pay-for-performance and the Quality and Outcomes Framework

CHAPTER 10

Pay-for-performance schemes in primary care: what have we learnt?

Stephen Peckham and Andrew Wallace

SUMMARY

Pay-for-performance (P4P) schemes have become increasingly popular with commissioners of primary care and other health services and this has generated questions about their effect on improving quality. In this chapter, we draw on relevant literature and primary research to reflect on how the Quality and Outcomes Framework has impacted on general practice in the United Kingdom, while reflecting upon the relationship between P4P schemes and quality improvement more generally. We argue that, although evidence for the effect of P4P on quality is limited, P4P schemes do have an effect on the behaviour of physicians and can lead to better clinical management of disease, but that there is cause for concern about their impact on the wider aspects of quality of care. We conclude that P4P schemes need to take more account of broader definitions of quality since, while schemes can have a positive impact on incentivised clinical processes, it is not clear that this translates into improving the experience and outcome of care for patients.

Key points
- P4P schemes are increasingly being used to enhance the quality of primary care provision.
- The relationship between P4P and primary care quality can be ill-defined and in tension.
- P4P schemes can change behaviour and improve disease management, but it is unclear whether they are improving care quality in a broader sense of patient experience, safety and effectiveness.
- The focus of many P4P schemes on clinical process should not be allowed to crowd out broader definitions of care quality improvement.

INTRODUCTION

There is increasing international interest in pay-for-performance (P4P) systems in primary care. Their introduction reflects concerns about three interlinked issues – variation in performance and quality, the emphasis on driving improvements in performance and ensuring high quality primary care.[1] This chapter briefly examines the current evidence on P4P schemes and the extent to which such schemes can contribute to quality in primary care services. We start by identifying key aspects of quality relevant to primary care and then examine the relationship between P4P schemes and quality criteria.

DEFINING QUALITY IN PRIMARY CARE

Primary care by its very nature is likely to encompass substantial variation in practice because of the nature of the delivery and organisation of care (e.g., different staff mixes and training levels) and also to external contextual factors (socio-demographic factors, geography, etc). In the United Kingdom, variation in practice standards have been observed over many years.[2] In 2004, the Government renegotiated the GP Contract incorporating a P4P element – the Quality and Outcomes Framework (QOF) – which would account for around 20–30% of practice income. The QOF financially rewards practices for the quality of care they deliver to patients across four domains: clinical, organisational, patient experience and extra services such as maternity and child health. As a recent survey by Schoen *et al.*[3] demonstrates, other P4P systems for primary care have been developed in a number of countries, although the degree to which financial incentives are employed to improve the quality of primary care varies. Primary care physicians in the United States (33%), Sweden (10%) and Norway (35%) are less likely to be receiving financial incentives, whereas primary care physicians in countries such as the United Kingdom (89%), the Netherlands (81%), New Zealand (80%), Italy (70%) and Australia (65%) are more likely to receive financial incentives.[4] The design of P4P schemes varies, but they tend to be based on clinical activity targets.

However, performance as a measure of quality depends upon what the performance standards are and how they are measured. Hogg *et al.* argue that the performance domain in such P4P schemes is divided into two main components: healthcare delivery and technical quality of clinical care.[5] This is an important distinction as most P4P systems focus on aspects of clinical care rather than including delivery systems. Giuffrida *et al.* also caution that it is important not to confuse performance indicators with health outcomes.[6] A key point is to examine the match between performance targets and those criteria generally seen as central to the provision of high-quality primary care.

There has been a longstanding debate about the nature of quality in healthcare services and, as Eddy argues, the science of quality measurement is still in its adolescence.[7] Defining quality is also complex and a number of different definitions have been developed over the years such as those of Donabedian[8] and Maxwell,[9] statements of quality such as those by the Royal College of General Practitioners on quality as excellence, or the Institute of Medicine, which defines quality as 'the degree to which health services for individuals and populations increase the likelihood of desired health outcomes and are consistent with current professional knowledge'.[10] All recognise that quality is a complex and multi-dimensional concept.[11,12] There is also a distinction to be made between a quality health service and quality care to individuals. This point is particularly relevant in examining quality in primary care, where Campbell *et al.* have argued that individual care is more important than broader health system measures of quality.[13] They offer their own definition of quality as 'whether individuals can access the health structures and processes of care, which they need and whether the care received is effective'. They focus on two aspects of individual care that they see as relevant to primary care – access and effectiveness. Reviews of primary care do demonstrate that these are the key aspects of care leading to improved health outcomes.[14,15] However, they do not identify quality in primary care in themselves. Too much emphasis on individual factors ignores key population aspects of primary care as identified by Starfield *et al.*, and studies demonstrate that there are no specific aspects of primary care that are associated uniformly with improved quality of care.[16,17]

There have been a number of attempts to define quality in primary care. The task is made more complex by the lack of any universal definition of primary care. As comparative international studies demonstrate, there are distinct differences between health systems as to what constitutes primary care let alone definitional complexities between terms such as family practice, general practice, primary medical and primary healthcare.[18,19] In the United Kingdom, primary care is frequently equated with general practice. However, care must be exercised in universalising both the definitions of quality and the impact of P4P.

Wilson *et al.* suggest that there are four broad areas upon which the performance of primary care, and general practice specifically, should be measured. These are equity, quality of clinical care, responsiveness to patients and efficiency.[20] Their review of practice suggested that UK practices score highly in all four domains although there have been recent concerns about a lack of support for self-care[21,22] and poor support for people with long-term conditions.[23] The fact that inequalities in health at a primary care level persist[24] also raises questions about whether general practice can retain this strong position.

Starfield identifies four unique features of primary care service: first contact access, person-focused care over time, comprehensiveness and coordination.[25] Hogg *et al.* suggest that other important aspects of primary care include patient-provider relationships as defined by communication, holistic care and an awareness of the patient's family and culture.[26] Primary care performance needs to be set within a broader structural environment that recognises the wider healthcare system, the practice context and the organisation of the practice. This reflects an increasing acceptance of the role of the healthcare delivery system including processes of governance and accountability, resource allocation and inter-relationships between primary care and other health and social care services.[27]

Furthermore, in a review of outcome indicators for primary care, Sans-Corralles *et al.* identified key attributes linked to patient satisfaction, health outcomes and cost of services provided.[28] They found that improved satisfaction and health outcomes were associated with continuity of care, patient-centred care, longer appointments and a good patient – doctor personal relationship. These factors were also associated with lower overall health costs. Continuity of care is consistently reported as a key attribute and quality indicator of good primary medical care (general practice/family medicine).[29]

However, studies on primary care show these attributes are often not uniformly attributable. Size of practice, practice population and the culture of the practice are all important factors related to the delivery of primary care and patient experiences and outcomes.[30] These influences on quality are less likely to be included in P4P schemes given their clinical focus despite the evidence highlighting them as key components of primary care performance and quality. Indeed, of particular interest is the way P4P schemes are starting to redefine how quality is conceptualised in practice. A number of recent articles reporting on P4P, especially in the United Kingdom, appear to equate quality with the P4P criteria.[31,32,33,34]

P4P AND QUALITY: WHAT IS THE EVIDENCE?

Despite some scepticism about the evidence base of the effectiveness of P4P schemes in improving quality,[35] recent systematic reviews[36,37] have concluded that P4P contracts do affect physician behaviour and increase the number of primary care services provided – although often in complex and limited ways.[38] The modest effects of financial incentives tend to be measured in the literature in relation to improvements in the management of chronic disease reflecting the focus on clinical processes found in most P4P schemes.[39] There are concerns that improvements in clinical process measures may not be reflected in better patient outcomes[40] and that not enough attention has been paid to linking financial incentives with sustainable quality improvements.[41] Nonetheless, the actual effect of financial incentives depends on factors such as the age and sex of physicians, previous experience of financial incentives, the uptake of continuing professional education, the type of payment method, the type and severity of the conditions targeted through incentives, the volume of activity and the location and type of organisation.[42]

A key concern that recurs in the literature is whether financial incentives generate dysfunctional physician behaviour[43] or negatively affect motivation,[44] particularly in light of well-established inverse care patterns at primary care level.[45] Some commentators have argued that there is a risk of neglecting resources of emotion, morality and trust, which are said to be a key part of the physician's professional repertoire.[46] Research with GPs in the United Kingdom revealed that they are anxious that 'biomedical' targets might undermine holistic, continuity of care of the 'whole person' and might mitigate against developing relationships with patients, as treatment is increasingly divided up by larger teams of health practitioners,[47] as practices seek to set up more efficient disease management systems and as GPs offload routine tasks to nursing staff.

There is evidence that physicians who work within incentive systems designed to reduce secondary care referral rates are anxious that their ability to deliver quality care for their patients could be compromised as they experience pressure to reduce referral rates.[48]

A further concern about the impact of externally structured incentives such as financial inducements is that they might 'crowd out' professional self-esteem and a sense of self-determination. However, it has been noted that there is an equal chance of a 'crowding in' effect if practitioners feel like they have some ownership of incentives.[49] Indeed, one study in the United Kingdom found that the QOF as an externally imposed system of incentives did not appear to damage the internal motivation of GPs.[50] The authors attributed this to the fact that the indicators within the QOF aligned with what GPs themselves considered good clinical care objectives. This could be because performance indicators in the QOF were negotiated with representatives of the profession itself, which ensured a degree of alignment of objectives and reduced the potential for decreased internal motivation.[51] A recent study suggested that GPs feel that, though professional autonomy has decreased and workload increased, they are paid more, their job satisfaction levels continue to improve and job pressures decrease under the QOF. GPs also report that they feel the QOF has had a more positive impact on quality of care than they initially thought.[52] Nonetheless, there is evidence that GPs remain anxious about the impact of external incentives on professional (internal) motivation.

Another potential problem created by an external financial incentive schemes is that they could lead to the neglect of those non-incentivised areas of care, which will continue to rely on the professionalism or moral motivation of GPs. There is some evidence of concern among GPs that un-incentivised areas like acute care, preventive care, care for specific groups like children or older people, patients with multiple co-morbidities would suffer as GPs chased targets. Indeed, a study found that, while quality of care for QOF-incentivised conditions improved substantially between 2003 and 2005, there was little or no improvement in non-incentivised quality indicators.[53] However, it has also been argued that this could be positively interpreted as GPs maintaining standards of care in these areas despite the lack of incentives and the time required to focus on QOF targets.[54]

Research conducted in the United States has found that the size and structure of incentives seems to be important in promoting effective physician activity. Incentives have to be large enough to influence behaviour[55] and designed in such a way that they cannot be gamed so as to reward both process and improved outcomes.[56] However, the size of incentive has also been found to be less of a factor in the use of care management processes for patients with chronic illnesses by 'physician organisations' than schemes that give public recognition for scoring well on quality of care measures, schemes that require 'physician organisations' to provide quality of care or outcomes data to outside organisations or those that reward high-quality scores with better contracts that assist in developing better organized quality provision.[57]

Questions continue to circulate about the likely individual and population health gain from P4P schemes. Evidence of physician activity does not always correspond to better health outcomes or broader definitions of quality.[58] The evidence of a relationship between incentive payments and health gain appears to be weak or mixed.[59] Furthermore, it is difficult to detect patterns from the diverse range of definitions of quality and the outcome measures used by researchers. The most common measure – mortality – may be unreliable because it is affected by wide range of factors and, as with other outcome measures, may be difficult to achieve or beyond the control of the physician or provider.[60] Some studies have called for a combination of process and outcome measures when structuring incentives.[61] It is technically challenging to connect performance targets with health gain. Most P4P schemes adopt a pragmatic approach and focus on processes (such as measuring blood pressure) and intermediate outcomes (controlled blood pressure), for which there is either evidence or professional consensus and that can be measured and rewarded. Treatment and secondary prevention are thus favoured over primary prevention and some conditions can be marginalised. In order to promote quality improvement, financial incentives need to operate alongside better resourced primary care organisations, a robust data infrastructure and closer physician and staff engagement in the design of quality interventions[62] in order to provide the capacity to 'leverage' substantive changes in performance.[63]

In the United Kingdom, the evidence as to whether the QOF rewards outputs that lead to good outcomes is contradictory. It demonstrates both that meeting certain QOF indicators might improve health outcomes in some areas[64] and a weak causal relationship between key clinical indicators and outcomes (*see* Chapter 4). There is some concern that the QOF may lead to an exacerbation of health inequalities by allowing GPs to 'game' the exception reporting system and exclude 'high risk' patients, or by not sufficiently rewarding the extra work required in delivering equal treatment to disadvantaged populations, maintaining inverse care patterns (*see* Chapter 6).[65] Inequities between population groups remain. For example, rates of statin prescribing in practices serving deprived populations are higher but prescribing volumes in practices with higher proportions of older people and minority ethnic groups are lower.[66]

CONCLUSIONS

In this chapter, we have reviewed key themes from the rapidly growing literature on P4P and raised concerns about the relationship between P4P and how we understand quality in primary care. The use of financial targets is effective in changing the behaviour and activities of practitioners (doctors and others). Such schemes, by setting targets, also have an impact on the range of activities undertaken by practitioners. Generally, the adoption of P4P schemes demonstrates that financial payments are a key incentive for increasing activity for clinical processes such as blood pressure measurement, cholesterol screening, statin prescribing and the measuring of blood sugar levels and body mass index. However, the implications for organisational aspects and patient care are less clear. P4P schemes have been criticised for not adequately addressing health outcomes and other aspects of patient-perceived quality. Although waiting times and access are measured in the QOF in the United Kingdom, these are not necessarily a priority for quality from a patient perspective. The literature on P4P tends to equate quality of primary care with clinical processes despite a substantial literature identifying other aspects of primary care as being important constituents of quality.[67,68,69]

Incentive payments may skew physician activity towards high-reward labour-intensive activities with relatively low-health benefits thereby marginalising non-incentivised areas. This potential for gaming may create a conflict of interest for physicians between maximising revenue and ensuring good quality care. Financial incentives may also distort care by encouraging a focus on individual measures for care management instead of a more integrated approach, particularly in areas of co-morbidity. In addition, the use of targets and financial incentives can have unintended consequences on practitioner behaviour such as goal displacement and rule following leading to the 'crowding out' of non-incentivised tasks. Thus, areas of clinical activity not included within P4P schemes become less important. Studies have also found that financial reward is not necessarily the main incentive for practitioners to engage in quality improvement. Although targets clearly deliver changes in behaviour, they can lead to goal misplacement in which rule-following becomes the means to the end. There is a need for intelligent and vigilant structuring of P4P schemes lest they lead to a narrowing of definitions of quality in primary care and restrict our focus to clinical process at a time when richer meanings of quality should be gaining currency.

ACKNOWLEDGEMENTS
We thank the editors for their constructive feedback and Kath Checkland for her insights into the impact of QOF on general practice.

REFERENCES
1. Doran T. Lesson from early experience with pay for performance. *Dis Manag Health Outcomes.* 2008; **16**(2): 69–77.
2. Majeed A, Bindman AB, Weiner JP. Use of risk adjustment in setting budgets and measuring performance in primary care II: advantages, disadvantages, and practicalities. *BMJ.* 2001; **323**: 607–10.

3. Schoen C, Osborn R, Doty MM, *et al.* A survey of primary care physicians in eleven countries, 2009: perspectives on care, costs, and experiences. *Health Aff (Millwood).* 2009; **28**: w1171–83.
4. Ibid.
5. Hogg W, Rowan M, Russell G, *et al.* Framework for primary care organization: the importance of a structural domain. *Qual Health Care.* 2008; **20**(5): 308–13.
6. Giuffrida A, Gosden T, Forland F, *et al.* Target payments in primary care: effects on professional practice and health care outcomes. *Cochrane Database Syst Rev.* 1999; **4**.
7. Eddy DM. Performance measurement: problems and solutions. *Health Aff.* 1998; **17**: 7–25.
8. Donabedian A. Explorations in quality assessment and monitoring. In: Donabedian A, editor. *The Definition of Quality and Approaches to its Assessment.* Vol. 1. Ann Arbor, MI: Health Administration Press; 1980.
9. Maxwell RJ. Quality assessment in health. *BMJ.* 1984; **288**: 1470–2.
10. Lohr K. *Medicare: A Strategy for Quality Assurance.* Washington, DC: National Academy Press; 1992.
11. Donabedian, op. cit.
12. Maxwell RJ. Dimensions of quality revisited: from thought to action. *Qual Health Care.* 1992; **1**: 171–7.
13. Campbell SM, Roland MO, Buetow SA. Defining quality of care. *Soc Sci Med.* 2000; **51**: 1611–25.
14. Ibid.
15. Starfield B, Shi L, Macinko J. Contribution of primary health care to health systems and health. *Milbank Q.* 2005; **83**(4): 457–502.
16. Ibid.
17. Campbell SM, Hann M, Hacker J, *et al.* Identifying predictors of high quality care in English general practice: observational study. *BMJ.* 2001; **323**: 1–6.
18. MacDonald J. *Primary Health Care: medicine in its place.* London: Earthscan; 1992.
19. Peckham S, Exworthy M. *Primary Care in the UK: policy, organisation and management.* Basingstoke: Palgrave; 2003.
20. Wilson T, Roland M, Ham C. The contribution of general practice and the general practitioner to NHS patients. *J R Soc Med.* 2006; **99**: 24–8.
21. Department of Health. *Public Attitudes to Self Care: Baseline Survey.* London: DH; 2005.
22. Coulter A. *Engaging Patients in their Healthcare.* Oxford: Picker Institute Europe; 2006.
23. Department of Health. *Self Care—A Real Choice, Self Care Support—A Real Option.* London: DH; 2005.
24. Wilson, Roland, Ham, op. cit.
25. Starfield B. *Primary Care: Balancing Health Needs, Services, and Technology.* New York: Oxford University Press; 1998.
26. Hogg, Rowan, Russell, *et al.*, op. cit.
27. Starfield, Shi, Macinko, op. cit.
28. Sans-Corralles M, Pujol-Ribera E, Gene-Badia J, *et al.* Family medicine attributes related to satisfaction, health and costs. *Fam Pract.* 2006; **23**: 308–16.
29. Saulz JW, Albedaiwi W. Interpersonal continuity of care and patient satisfaction: a critical review. *Ann Fam Med* 2004; **2**: 445–51.

30. Campbell, Hann, Hacker, *et al.*, op. cit.

31. Roland M, Campbell S, Bailey N, *et al.* Financial incentives to improve the quality of care in the UK: predicting the consequences of change. *Prim Health Care Res Dev.* 2006; **7**: 18–26.

32. Whalley D, Gravelle H, Sibbald B. Effect of the new contract on GPs' working lives and perceptions of quality of care: a longitudinal survey. *Br J Gen Pract.* 2008; **58**: 8–14.

33. McElduff P, Lyratzopoulos G, Edwards R, *et al.* Will changes in primary care improve health outcomes? Modelling the impact of financial incentives introduced to improve quality of care in the UK. *Qual Saf Health Care.* 2004; **13**: 191–7.

34. Campbell S, Reeves D, Kontopantelis E, *et al.* Effects of pay for performance on quality of care in England. *N Engl J Med.* 2009; **361**(4): 368–78.

35. Rosenthal M, Frank R. What is the empirical basis for paying for quality in health care? *Med Care Res Rev.* 2006; **63**(2): 135–57.

36. Chaix-Couturier C, Durand-Zaleski I, Jolly D, *et al.* Effects of financial incentives on medical practice: results from a systematic review of the literature and methodological issues. *Int J Qual Health Care.* 2000; **12**(2): 133–42.

37. Gosden T, Forland F, Kristiansen IS, *et al.* Impact of payment method on behaviour of primary care physicians: a systematic review. *J Health Serv Res Policy.* 2001; **6**(1): 44–55.

38. Christianson J, Leatherman S, Sutherland K. *Financial Incentives, Healthcare Providers and Quality Improvements: a review of the evidence.* London: The Health Foundation; 2008.

39. Chung S, Palaniappan LP, Trujillo LM, *et al.* Effect of physician-specific pay for performance incentives in a large group practice. *Am J Manag Care.* 2010; **16**(2): 35–42.

40. Glickman S, Peterson E. Innovative health reform models: pay for performance initiatives. *Am J Manag Care.* 2009; **15**: S300–5.

41. McNamara P. Quality-based payment: six case examples. *Int J Qual Health Care.* 2005; **17**(4): 357–62.

42. Chaix-Couturier, Durand-Zaleski, Jolly, *et al.*, op. cit.

43. Gravelle H, Sutton M, Ma A. *Doctor Behaviour Under a Pay for Performance Contract: further evidence from the Quality and Outcomes Framework.* CHE Research Paper. York: Centre for Health Economics, University of York; 2008.

44. McDonald R, Harrison S, Checkland K, *et al.* Impact of financial incentives on clinical autonomy and internal motivation in primary care: an ethnographic study. *BMJ.* 2007; **334**: 1357–60.

45. McLean G, Sutton M, Guthrie B. Deprivation and the quality of primary care services: evidence of the persistence of the inverse care law from the UK Quality and Outcomes Framework. *J Epidemiol Community Health.* 2006; **60**(11): 917–22.

46. Harrison S, Smith C. Trust and moral motivation: redundant resources in health and social care? *Policy Polit.* 2004; **32**(3): 371–86.

47. Marshall M, Harrison S. It's about more than money: financial incentives and internal motivation. *Qual Saf Health Care.* 2005; **14**: 4–5.

48. Chung, Palaniappan, Trujillo, *et al.*, op. cit.

49. McDonald, Harrison, Checkland, *et al.*, op. cit.

50. McDonald, Harrison, Checkland, *et al.*, op. cit.

51. Roland, Campbell, op. cit.

52. Whalley, Gravelle, Sibbald, op. cit.

53. Steel N, Maisey S, Clarke A, *et al.* Quality of clinical care and targeted incentive payments: an observational study. *Br J Gen Pract.* 2007; **58**(539): 449–54.

54. Roland M. The Quality and Outcomes Framework: too early for a final verdict. *Br J Gen Pract.* 2007; **57**: 525–7.

55. Town R, Kane R, Johnson P, *et al.* Economic incentives and physicians' delivery of preventive care. *Am J Prev Med.* 2005; **28**(2): 234–40.

56. Petersen L, Woodward L, Urech T, *et al.* Does pay-for-performance improve the quality of health care? *Ann Intern Med.* 2006; **14**: 265–72.

57. Casalino L, Gillies R, Shortell S. External incentives, information technology and organised processes to improve health care quality for patients with chronic diseases. *JAMA.* 2003; **22**(29): 434–41.

58. Gosden, Forland, Kristiansen, *et al.*, op. cit.

59. Christianson, Leatherman, Sutherland, op. cit.

60. Gosden, Forland, Kristiansen, *et al.*, op. cit.

61. National Audit Office. *NHS Pay Modernisation: new contracts for general practice services in England.* London: TSO; 2008.

62. Chung, Palaniappan, Trujillo, *et al.*, op. cit.

63. Custers T, Hurley J, Klazinga N, *et al.* Selecting effective incentive structures in health care: a decision framework to support health care purchasers in finding the right incentives to drive performance. *BMC Health Serv Res.* 2009; **8**: 66.

64. McElduff, Lyratzopoulos, Edwards, *et al.*, op. cit.

65. Ashworth M, Lloyd D, Smith R, *et al.* Social deprivation and statin prescribing: a cross sectional analysis using data from the new general practitioner Quality and Outcomes Framework. *J Public Health.* 2006; **29**(1): 40–7.

66. Spooner A, Chapple A, Roland M. What makes British general practitioners take part in a quality improvement scheme? *J Health Serv Res Policy.* 2001; **6**(3): 145–50.

67. Hogg, Rowan, Russell, *et al.*, op. cit.

68. Giuffrida, Gosden, Forland, *et al.*, op. cit.

69. Eddy, op. cit.

CHAPTER 11

An international perspective on the basis of pay-for-performance

Barbara Starfield and Dee Mangin

SUMMARY

The Quality and Outcomes Framework (QOF) is intended to bring the best scientific evidence to bear on primary care practice. However, the evidence base suffers from a variety of weaknesses, including particularly its attention to only a small set of problems in primary care, the absence of an evidence base for dealing with patients' problems as they experience them, the lack of generalisability of the evidence to primary care practice and biases and flaws in the evidence base itself.

The QOF has resulted in an increase in measuring the measurable and has proven again that physicians will do what they are paid to do. It has provided a mechanism for paying primary care physicians what they are worth. However, there is no evidence that what has been valued is the most valuable in terms of health. The questions remain in an increasingly loud silence about the costs and opportunity costs of the distortions that occur in individual care as a result.

An extraordinary amount of money has been spent on this system with no evidence of improvement in health outcomes of the scale that might be expected. The question that must be asked of all national level structural changes is not whether using money in this way has an effect, but rather is this the best use of this money? In the face of little evidence for the model chosen for the QOF, there is evidence for other indicators of the attributes of a primary care system most likely to improve health outcomes.[1]

The opportunity costs lie in the railroading of a disease-based model for understanding patient suffering, treatment effects and the nature of 'good care'. This threatens a transformation of education into simply training that will obscure critical thinking among physicians about the strengths, weaknesses and biases of the science they apply; erect barriers to wisdom and judgement in the application of treatments; and provide no opportunity to reflect on their own practice and assess the nature of the effects of the treatments they give.

One of the fundamental questions around initiatives designed to 'improve care' centres around the distinction between variation in practice that reflects poor care and variation that represents the complex relationships among the heterogeneity of patients, patterns of suffering and the effects of treatments beyond a simplistic licensed disease indication. The challenge for the future is to develop an innovative system that promotes and supports care, which is informed by the best medical science, yet provides informed options for primary care physicians and patients to choose alternatives. A rational system would provide for flexibility and responsiveness in applying evidence from partial statistical lives to complex individual lives. To be useful, any strategy for improving the health outcomes in primary care must include a mechanism for detecting unintended consequences, adverse events, worsened health and insufficient cost effectiveness.

Key points
- The QOF and patient-centred medicine are often at odds.
- Inadequacies and commercial bias in the creation of evidence make the scientific basis of the QOF questionable.
- The framework for the QOF does not align well with the scope of primary care, making its basis as a tool for quality measurement questionable.
- The extent of impact of the QOF on health outcomes and on equity of health outcomes needs examination.
- Alternative modes of improving patient care may be better than the QOF.
- Attention to the resolution of patients' problems is an important aim of quality improvement activities.

INTRODUCTION
The chapters in this volume provide a balanced perspective on the Quality and Outcomes Framework (QOF), as it has played out in the British context. It is clear that there have been many successes, not the least of which is the apparent widespread acceptance of the process by practitioners and improvement in their 'performance'. However, there also appears to be general agreement that there is no evidence that health has improved, no understanding of the meaning of exception reporting and its relevance to patients' care, no indication that what is measured is either most important to measure or generalisable beyond what is measured, no sense that the evidence on which it is based is clinically valid and no evidence that it is the best approach to improving care among the alternatives that might be available. It is apparent that there have been some unintended consequences.

All of the chapters in this book seem to agree that there is little relationship between clinical quality as measured by proxy indicators for a limited number of specific diseases and outcomes of care as measured by improvements in health. Kordowicz and Ashworth raise the question of whether pay-for-performance (as in the QOF) may lead to a misrepresentation of the epidemiology of primary care practice but without directly questioning the validity of a disease-by-disease approach to quality of care. Peckham and Wallace raise the important issue of the crowding out of professional esteem by rote management, a subject well treated by Iliffe in his book.[2] Lester and Campbell point out that the QOF was justified on the basis of variations in costs and practices, the need to reduce high-profile malpractice, to take advantage of 'the art of the possible' based on research findings, and the opportunity to redress the underfunding of the incomes of primary care practitioners with the choice of indicators dictated by internal coherence within clinical domains that are relevant to primary care practice. Checkland and Harrison ask whether the QOF meets patients' needs and raise the possibility that team activities will become increasingly, biomedically oriented. The possibility that practice dynamics might be changed by the increasing use of nurses to control adherence is a real but largely unrecognised concern. The contribution by Dixon and Khachatryan reflects on the lack of recognition of and possible conflicts between clinical issues, a focus on inequalities, cost effectiveness, quality and health outcomes and stresses that it is not clear whether reductions in inequities in performance translate into better equity in health. They are also concerned that considerable overuse may be resulting from the focus on 'doing things'.

Collectively, the authors of these chapters appropriately address the issue of exception reporting; they might have asked why there has been no systematic study of the reasons why certain patients are excepted or of the impact of target levels recommended by the General Medical Services (GMS) contract, which differ from those recommended by the National Institute for Health and Clinical Excellence and the British Hypertension Society,[3] and they make no judgement on the wisdom of paying for time rather than for benefit.[4] Citing a study of benefits from adherence to diabetes guidelines, they do not address the nature of these benefits: are they definitive or are they just proxy health indicators?[5]

As it is surprising that none of the contributions have questioned the rationale for the choice of indicators or the focus on a particular set of diseases, the purpose of this paper is to address the justification for the choice of indicators and open a discussion of possible alternatives for improving quality of and payment for primary care.

PATIENT-CENTRED CARE AND GUIDELINES

Patient-centred care is based on values that often conflict with clinical practice guidelines. Thoughtful physicians recognise that focusing on guidelines interferes with patient-centredness, because they sometimes seem to be at cross-purposes. Patient-centred care means '…healthcare that establishes a partnership … to ensure that decisions respect patients' wants, needs and preferences, and that patients have the education and support they need to make decisions and participate in their own care'[6] or, alternatively, care that '…is designed and delivered to address the health-care needs and preferences of patients so that healthcare is appropriate and cost-effective'.[7] Primary care physicians devoted to patient-centred care may feel uneasy when such care appears to contravene standard guidelines. In contrast, healthcare funders and administrators often see systems that embrace and incentivise guidelines and targets (such as the QOF) as proxies for 'high-quality care', so that it is possible to provide care that is financially rewarded for being measurably 'good'. However, 'measurably good' often means meaningfully worse for individual patients. The reasons for this dilemma are best understood in these terms: the nature of evidence, the nature of patients and the nature of individuals.

The nature of evidence

Almost everyone agrees that it is a good idea to assemble and make accessible the best possible evidence and relevant expertise to aid physicians and patients in making decisions about interventions. Everything beyond this is controversial. Guidelines translated into targets such as the QOF have been held as representing a standard of evidence which, when followed, demonstrates practice of evidence-based medicine (EBM). In examining how guidelines and targets fit within the paradigm of EBM, it is apparent that there is little if any justification for assuming that pay for adhering to guidelines improves health status, not because providing financial incentives does not improve 'performance' but because improving performance has an unknown relationship to improving health.

The original concept of EBM that Sackett enshrined was 'the integration of best research evidence with clinical expertise and patient values'.[8] Guidelines reflect the state of available evidence, but this is disconnected from the context of patient care, especially the constellation of an individual patient's health needs and preferences. Despite the limitations in both internal and external validity of clinical trials on which guidelines are based, the adoption of practice guidelines removes any doubt about the scientific basis of guideline-directed medical interventions and thus reduces the likelihood of learning from variability in outcomes in different populations. It takes a seasoned practitioner with an inquiring mind to understand that medicine is an inexact science and that guidelines and targets do not necessarily improve outcomes of interventions.

Protocol-driven medicine has been based on a model of quality that has its roots in the production line efficiency models developed in Japan where the car that was produced at the end of every line was perfect and identical. It has led to a single disease focus in delivery and measurement of care, which aims, like the production line, at standardised delivery of evidence-based care under the assumption that improved health outcomes will result. Clinical guidelines focus on disease management, not on patients' patterns of morbidity within which diseases are inseparable. QOF shifts the focus from ill health in patients to an abstract notion of single disease prevention and management, which is the same in everyone diagnosed with them. Even without overt co-morbidity, patients experience illnesses differently, depending on their biological, social and environmental contexts. This variation increases as co-morbidity becomes the rule.

Only a few interventions are experienced uniformly, with few harms and with evident benefits, in everyone: e.g., immunization, handwashing and measuring blood pressure in both arms,[9] for which adherence to guidelines and targets is unequivocally appropriate. Where unquestioned adherence to guideline-based interventions is not appropriate is in the ongoing care of people with changing health needs, i.e., in primary care.

The idea of guidelines implies a great deal more certainty than is warranted. In the United Kingdom, only about a quarter of the QOF indicators are based on sound evidence.[10] Even where most is known – cardiovascular disease – a recent review of American College of Cardiology (ACC) and American Heart Association (AHA) guidelines showed that, of 2711 recommendations, only one in 10 are based on strong evidence while half are based on level C evidence (i.e., consensus), where consensus may be influenced by inclusions of individuals and groups with conflicts of interest.[11] Moreover, knowledge in medicine is often short lived. Many patients take aspirin for primary prevention of cardiovascular disease, but recent research indicates that the risk benefit ratio is not favourable for use as primary prevention.[12,13] Reaching control targets for HbA1c specified in most current guidelines will result in more rather than fewer patient deaths.[14]

Evidence is increasingly commercially constructed in a way that is likely to overstate benefits and underestimate (or even hide) the harmful effects of treatments. Half of efficacy and two-thirds of harm outcomes are incompletely reported, and two-thirds of trials have a primary outcome that was changed.[15] Results and conclusions are biased in favour of the funding company's drug. Papers are often ghost written, and publication decisions are influenced by subtle commercial interests.[16] Trial data are not available for public scrutiny.[17] Virtually all 'evidence' is generated in highly selected populations and therefore does not reflect most primary care settings. Populations needing or using multiple medications are those most likely to be those excluded from the clinical trials.

An average of four-fifths of the members of guideline development groups have a conflict of interest, mostly with the companies making drugs related to the guideline.[18] Using medications to reach targets while improving the intermediate 'numbers' can worsen real health outcomes.[19,20,21]

The nature of patients

The landscape of primary care is an uncertain one; 40% of consultations have no diagnostic label. The second important characteristic of the primary care landscape is co-morbidity. Patients seen in primary care most often have multiple coexisting illnesses. A 70-year-old woman with three chronic diseases and two risk factors, if guidelines were followed, would be prescribed 19 different doses of 12 different medicines at five different times of day.[22] More importantly, there are 10 possibilities for significant drug interactions, either with other medicines or with other diseases.[23] This prescriber would be rated as a good physician using single disease measures, whereas the physician using wisdom and judgement in avoiding polypharmacy would be rated low on adherence.

The therapeutic imperative provided by single disease guidelines drives polypharmacy – probably one of the greatest but most invisible threats to health in ageing populations. The majority of older people take more than five medications with the median number around seven.[24,25,26] In 1990, adverse events were estimated to be the third leading cause of all deaths in the United States.[27] The risk of hospitalisation due to inappropriate medication use in older adults is estimated to be around 17%, six times that in the general population. The risk of an adverse drug reaction rises strikingly with the number of medicines taken.[28]

The nature of individuals
Personalised advice that is evidence-informed in the context of peoples' lives is the essence of primary care. Treatment must relate to outcomes that are important to the patient. The medical model decides what diseases are of highest priority,[29] but there are other priorities.[30] A focus on single disease-based guideline adherence can override respect for patient autonomy and patient welfare.

The use of statins to reduce heart disease deaths cannot be the main aim of treatment, which must always be to maximise overall functioning while, at the same time, maximising the overall duration of life for those who wish it. There is evidence that using statins for prevention at older ages simply shifts the cause of morbidity and mortality without any overall improvement in quality or quantity of life.[31] Many patients fear the manner of their dying more than death itself and have quite clear preferences about what is a 'good death'. Despite the distressing nature of some cardiac deaths, many people regard coronary heart disease as a 'good way to go' in old age. Using a single disease lens, we may be selecting for another cause of death unknowingly and certainly without the patient's informed consent.

There is no intervention without a possible unintended effect. Sometimes 'not doing' is the mark of good care because the treatment would do more harm than good, or because adding another treatment would do more harm than good. Guidelines create a therapeutic imperative that produces technological brinkmanship when there is no guideline for deciding when enough is enough.[32] Defining the experience of health must always take precedence over disease care, no matter what disease experts maintain are high priorities for health system attention.

The challenge for the future is to develop an innovative system that promotes and supports care that is informed by the best medical science yet provides informed options for general practitioners and patients to choose alternatives. A more rational system would provide for flexibility and responsiveness in applying evidence from partial statistical lives to complex individual lives. Such a system will not leave patients wondering 'are you doing this for me doctor, or am I doing it for you?'

ALTERNATIVE STRATEGIES TO ACHIEVING HIGH QUALITY AND PATIENT-CENTRED CARE

Are there alternatives for rewarding care that is both clinically relevant and patient-centred? We think so and offer the following ideas. Currently, practitioners learn to focus on patients' problems in addition to their own medically defined diagnoses. They have no incentive to remember patients' problems once they have made a diagnosis. Because we know that agreement between patients and practitioners is associated with a greater likelihood of improvement in patients' health,[33] quality efforts should focus more on adequate recognition of patients' problems, the extent to which patients and practitioners agree on what the patients' problems are and the degree to which these problems resolve or improve over time with medical and other interventions.

Increased survival over the 20th century and increasingly earlier diagnoses mean that patients with single diseases are no longer the norm. Almost everyone has co-morbidity – at least in adulthood; this pattern of co-morbidity is known as 'multimorbidity'.[34] Everyone can be categorized by their unique pattern of multimorbidity; different population groups have different patterns of multimorbidity.[35] Quality efforts must shift to reducing the impact of multimorbidity on life course events, on disability, and on burdens of care-inducing polypharmacy, and to understanding which types of interventions are more efficient and most equitable. Mechanisms are available to facilitate data collection on multimorbidity (www.acg.jhu); these can be used in efforts targeted at managing and developing new strategies for quality assessment and promotion. Assessment of patient-focused (not disease-focused) care will be aided by new mechanisms of characterizing health outcomes, such as by use of the International Classification of Functioning.[36]

Ongoing and life-long learning is the major impetus to quality improvement. Practitioners should be part of a system-wide effort to engage them in studying their own practices with regard to degree of patient improvement in health, variations in outcomes across their patients and patient populations, occurrence of unintended effects of treatments (including adverse ones) and in supporting acceptable deviations from 'standard' practices. If practitioners are not actively engaged in examining their own practices and the effects and adverse effects of the treatments they give and stimulated to ask questions about what they do, the only alternative is paying them to do what imperfect 'evidence' says they should be doing. Rational thinking dictates that the latter is decidedly suboptimal in terms of the goals of health systems.

REFERENCES

1. Starfield B, Shi L, Macinko J. Contribution of primary care to health systems and health. *Milbank Q.* 2005; **83**(3): 457–502.
2. Iliffe S. *From General Practice to Primary Care.* Oxford, UK: Oxford University Press; 2008.
3. National Institute for Health and Clinical Excellence. *Management of Hypertension in Adults in Primary Care.* London, UK: National Institute for Health and Clinical Excellence; 2006.
4. Gervas J, Starfield B, Heath I. Is clinical prevention better than cure? *Lancet.* 2008; **372**(9654): 1997–9.
5. Millett C, Saxena S, Ng A, *et al.* Socio-economic status, ethnicity and diabetes management: an analysis of time trends using the health survey for England. *J Public Health.* 2007; **29**(4): 413–19.
6. Hurtado MP, Swift EK, Corrigan J; Institute of Medicine Committee on the National Quality Report on Health Care Delivery and Board on Health Care Services. *Envisioning the National Health Care Quality Report.* Washington, DC: National Academies Press; 2001.
7. International Alliance of Patients' Organizations. *Declaration on Patient-Centred Healthcare.* London, UK; 2006. Available at: www.patientsorganizations.org/show article.pl?id=712&n=312 (accessed 17 October 2008).
8. Sackett DL, Rosenberg WM, Gray JA, *et al.* Evidence based medicine: what it is and what it isn't. *BMJ.* 1996; **312**(7023): 71–2.
9. Potts M, Prata N, Walsh J, *et al.* Parachute approach to evidence based medicine. *BMJ.* 2006; **333**(7570): 701–3.
10. Campbell SM, Roland MO, Shekelle PG, *et al.* Development of review criteria for assessing the quality of management of stable angina, adult asthma, and non-insulin dependent diabetes mellitus in general practice. *Qual Health Care.* 1999; **8**(1): 6–15.
11. Tricoci P, Allen JM, Kramer JM, *et al.* Scientific evidence underlying the ACC/AHA clinical practice guidelines. *JAMA.* 2009; **301**(8): 831–41.
12. Baigent C, Blackwell L, Collins R, *et al.*; Antithrombotic Trialists' (ATT) Collaboration. Aspirin in the primary and secondary prevention of vascular disease: collaborative meta-analysis of individual participant data from randomised trials. *Lancet.* 2009; **373**(9678): 1849–60.
13. Berger JS. Aspirin as preventive therapy in patients with asymptomatic vascular disease. *JAMA.* 2010; **303**(9): 880–2.
14. Gerstein HC, Miller ME, Byington RP, *et al.*; Action to Control Cardiovascular Risk in Diabetes Study Group. Effects of intensive glucose lowering in type 2 diabetes. *N Engl J Med.* 2008; **358**(24): 2545–59.
15. Chan AW, Hrobjartsson A, Haahr MT, *et al.* Empirical evidence for selective reporting of outcomes in randomized trials: comparison of protocols to published articles. *JAMA.* 2004; **291**(20): 2457–65.

16. Rising K, Bacchetti P, Bero L. Reporting bias in drug trials submitted to the Food and Drug Administration: review of publication and presentation. *PLoS Med.* 2008; 5(11): e217; discussion e217.

17. Godlee F. We want raw data, now. *BMJ.* 2009; **339**: b5405.

18. Choudhry NK, Stelfox HT, Detsky AS. Relationships between authors of clinical practice guidelines and the pharmaceutical industry. *JAMA.* 2002; **287**(5): 612–17.

19. Gerstein, Miller, Byington, *et al., op. cit.*

20. Barter PJ, Caulfield M, Eriksson M, *et al.* Effects of torcetrapib in patients at high risk for coronary events. *N Engl J Med.* 2007; **357**(21): 2109–22.

21. Anderson GL, Limacher M, Assaf AR, *et al.* Effects of conjugated equine estrogen in postmenopausal women with hysterectomy: the Women's Health Initiative randomized controlled trial. *JAMA.* 2004; **291**(14): 1701–12.

22. Boyd CM, Darer J, Boult C, *et al.* Clinical practice guidelines and quality of care for older patients with multiple comorbid diseases: implications for pay for performance. *JAMA.* 2005; **294**(6): 716–24.

23. Ibid.

24. Bon Hoem J, Kerse N, Scahill S, *et al.* Use of aspirin and statins for cardiovascular risk reduction in New Zealand: the residential care story. *J Prim Health Care.* 2009; **1**(3): 184–9.

25. Oakley Browne MA, Wells JE, Scott KM. *Te Rau Hinengaro: The New Zealand Mental Health Survey.* Wellington, NZ: Ministry of Health; 2006.

26. Kaufman DW, Kelly JP, Rosenberg L, *et al.* Recent patterns of medication use in the ambulatory adult population of the United States: the Slone survey. *JAMA.* 2002; **287**(3): 337–44.

27. Starfield B. Is US health really the best in the world? *JAMA.* 2000; **284**(4): 483–5.

28. Col N, Fanale JE, Kronholm P. The role of medication noncompliance and adverse drug reactions in hospitalizations of the elderly. *Arch Intern Med.* 1990; **150**(4): 841–5.

29. Institute of Medicine Committee on Quality of Health Care in America. *Crossing the Quality Chasm: a New Health System for the 21st century.* Washington, DC: National Academies Press; 2001.

30. Loeppke R, Taitel M, Richling D, *et al.* Health and productivity as a business strategy. *J Occup Environ Med.* 2007; **49**(7): 712–21.

31. Mangin D, Sweeney K, Heath I. Preventive health care in elderly people needs rethinking. *BMJ.* 2007; **335**(7614): 285–7.

32. Callahan D. *The Troubled Dream of Life.* Washington, DC: Georgetown University Press; 2000.

33. Starfield B. Primary care and equity in health: the importance to effectiveness and equity of responsiveness to peoples' needs. *Humanity Soc.* 2009; **33**(1–2): 56–73.

34. Valderas JM, Starfield B, Sibbald B, *et al.* Defining comorbidity: implications for understanding health and health services. *Ann Fam Med.* 2009; **7**(4): 357–63.

35. Starfield B, Weiner JP, Mumford L, *et al.* Ambulatory care groups: a categorization of diagnoses for research and management. *Health Serv Res.* 1991; **26**(1): 53–74.

36. World Health Organization. *International Classification of Functioning, Disability, and Health.* Geneva, Switzerland: World Health Organization; 2001.

CHAPTER 12

The Quality and Outcomes Framework: triumph of evidence or tragedy for personal care?

Steve Gillam and A Niroshan Siriwardena

SUMMARY

In this final chapter, we reflect on the contributions to this book and the ongoing work of those developing and researching the Quality and Outcomes Framework (QOF). We do not presume to provide a final verdict on the QOF. Indeed, any judgement will need to balance a nuanced evaluation of health gains against assessment of its costs, some of which are only now emerging and many of which are hard to describe let alone quantify.

It is hard to argue against the QOF's benefits to individuals – the reductions in morbidity and mortality, the suffering that has already been prevented. The question is not whether the QOF has had an effect, but rather concerns its cost effectiveness. Thus far, for the money spent, its health benefits appear unspectacular. We explore reasons for the QOF's limited health impact. We examine unintended consequences and ways of mitigating these. Finally, we look forward to a QOF-informed – if not yet QOFless – future.

HEALTHCARE GAINS

The main positive effects of the Quality and Outcomes Framework (QOF) have been relatively modest improvements in the quality of care measured and slight reductions in disparities between socioeconomic groups. Clearly, there has been improved recording, particularly in clinical areas and indicators newly conceived as part of the QOF. In the majority of cases, upward trends in clinical indicators were in line with increases that might have been predicted on the basis of secular or underlying movement before the introduction of the QOF.

It is easy to downplay these advances. Many of the health gains will be longer term, and it should not be forgotten that the benefits of more structured chronic disease management and extensive computerisation can spill over to other fields of practice activity. There is evidence that this has happened, more so for disease groups targeted by the QOF, but to a lesser extent in untargeted areas.[1] There have also been other positive, indirect effects of the QOF on practice organisation and the workforce, e.g., diversification of nurse roles.

LIMITATIONS

Our contributors have drawn attention to several factors impairing the QOF's population health impact. First, the process of 'exception reporting' reduces the public health effectiveness of population targets. On average, almost 7% of patients in England are excluded from public health targets such as achievement of serum cholesterol of <5 mmol/L. Second, targets are not set at 100%, albeit for good practical reasons. However, targets set at 70% for blood pressure control or cholesterol control in coronary heart disease further exclude 30% of patients from these public health targets. Thus, in combination with exception reporting, targets may shift the focus of the practice away from harder to reach patients, in exchange for more efficient achievement of results. More fundamentally, payment for adhering to guidelines cannot be assumed to improve health status, regardless of whether it improves 'performance'.

Starfield and Mangin point to the dangers of incentivising practice on evidence, which may be commercially constructed. For example, there is evidence of rising prescription rates for antidepressants[2] and statins[3,4] sometimes without evidence of improvement in proxy outcomes.[5] Even when performance appears to have improved, emerging evidence can reveal adverse effects of treating to target such as the recent evidence on the detrimental impact of over-tight control of blood glucose in type 2 diabetes mellitus.[6] Such unintended clinical consequences can sometimes, but not always, be anticipated. They require the processes for approval of new indicators or the disposal of old ones to be fast moving and flexible. To describe the QOF not so much as a pay-for-performance system, but as a 'pay-for-reporting' system misses the point.[7] The QOF's evidence base will only ever be partial.

COSTS

All contributors agree that the QOF has resulted in an increase in measuring the measurable, but the evidence on cost effectiveness is sparse. A current estimate puts the costs per additional record for each indicator at £50 (£25 per record if spill over effects are included).[8] When we consider that some recording relates to intermediate outcomes, recent evidence suggests that indicators in some domains may have been cost-effective.[9] However, there were a number of limitations in this evidence including lack of inclusion of costs for administration, unintended consequences or other services not provided as a result of the QOF. More sophisticated modelling is therefore required to clarify the overall cost effectiveness of the QOF. It is too early to assess the extent to which the supposed gains are illusory or whether their true costs are likely to be higher than current estimates. The opportunity costs are, by any reckoning, considerable; £1 billion per year might have been better spent on tobacco control or other public health initiatives. Could some of the gains have been delivered by other staff in other ways?

CHANGING ROLES, CHANGING PRACTICE

Simon and Morton provide intriguing insights into how QOF feels in day-to-day practice. With the entrepreneurial dynamism characteristic of UK general practice, practice teams have been swift to adapt to the imperatives of the QOF. However, a cursory glance through their '10 points' also betrays the extent to which core practice activities have been distorted around the QOF. For many practices, clinical governance and the QOF have become synonymous. Quality of care is narrowly focused on QOF domains and indicators to the exclusion of other areas for practice development, innovation and quality improvement.

Reassuringly, research has thus far found little evidence of clear cut gaming. However, there are no grounds for complacency. Research, including some as yet unpublished,[10] suggests clustering of blood pressure recordings below the upper systolic threshold in a manner that does not reflect the normal distribution of this variable.[11] While practices have frequently over-achieved in many areas, this is unsurprising as the individual practitioner may not be aware of his/her own practice's performance.

Several contributions illustrate the 'law' of unintended policy consequences: in this instance, the transformation of the primary care workforce and labour market. Greater specialisation among practice nurses has, in turn, promoted extension of the role of other cadres such as healthcare assistants in some practices. New roles and hierarchies have been created and accepted within practices. Practice staff have seen their roles expanded in the past, as now, but have not always shared the financial benefits, which may explain loss of motivation and demoralisation among some staff.[12,13]

The transition to a nurse-led primary care system is being accelerated by QOF in other ways. Since 1997 and the introduction of personal medical services, it has been possible and indeed advantageous for practices to employ salaried practitioners. QOF has hastened the stratification of medical roles. Salaried doctors and nurses with special interests are increasingly being seen as a more cost-efficient option when senior medical members of the primary health team need to be replaced.[14] Ultimately, this has contributed to the opening up of the primary care market to private providers. The exigencies of the market may over time drive the numbers of more expensive general practitioner (GP) principals down with the negative consequence of limiting the potential for career advancement for doctors entering general practice.

WHAT DO HEALTH PROFESSIONALS THINK?

Doctors and nurses are divided in their views on the QOF. While acknowledging that it may have improved quality of care and team-working in some areas, many are concerned about the depersonalising impact of the 'box-ticking culture', the intrusive impact of computerised prompts, and the move away from person-focused care and continuity. This ambivalence is partly explained by the threat of science devaluing the art of medicine embodied in the concept of the 'indeterminacy/ technicality ratio', where 'technicality' refers to scientific evidence and rationality whereas 'indeterminacy' is synonymous with uncertainty and individualisation.[15]

The development of evidence-based medicine has enabled the specialised knowledge of general practice to be deconstructed into its component parts, rationalised, codified and developed into guidelines, protocols and clinical indicators where the tasks defined may be carried out by others. The technicality of evidence-based care, by promoting the rationalisation of knowledge enhances general practice from the perspective of peers and patients.

Indeterminacy or uncertainty is a double-edged sword. Clinicians' uncertainty about diagnosis or management of their patient's condition does not usually enhance the patient's opinion of their doctor; it may even have an adverse effect on health outcomes.[16] If the patient's knowledge is equal to the doctor's, then the doctor becomes less useful or even irrelevant. Alternatively, the art of managing uncertainty is a positive asset to the GP when tacit knowledge and experience of the patient contribute to diagnosis and individualising care.[17] Where many treatment options exist, with similar outcomes, the doctor's skill in eliciting patient preferences allows the exercise of judgement in the grey zones of medicine.[18]

Many practitioners remain sceptical about the evidence base supporting new indicators, particularly when they have weak[19] or demonstrably negative consequences on care.[20] Others feel that the QOF is reducing continuity of care and promoting an overly mechanistic approach to chronic disease management, in which 'medicine by numbers' reduces clinical practice to a series of dichotomised decisions and reinforces a reductionist view of quality.

WHAT DO PATIENTS WANT?

Remarkably, little is known of what of those on the receiving end, including those of different age, sex, cultural background or clinical condition make of these changes.

This is a salutary reminder that what patients' experience of changing care is little understood and what users want and need remains an ongoing challenge to health professionals and services. The QOF has certainly changed the nature of medical discourse. What would Byrne and Long make of today's consultation transcripts?[21]

Computer-based templates categorising complaints into codes are embodying a biomedical rather than holistic approach. The 'McDonaldisation' of general practice as patients with multiple pathologies pass down various clinic-based production lines leaves little room for the deeper professional relationships patients want.[22]

Patricia Wilkie argues that 'what patients want from general practice is quality care given by a competent professional who is up-to-date, who knows the patient and who involves the patient in decision-making'. Measurably good can indeed mean meaningfully worse for individual patients. Interpersonal care and continuity are neglected within the current formula and need to be addressed.[23] Some aspects of care such as good access are not fully identified by current experience indicators.[24]

The QOF has begun another revolution in the assessment of primary healthcare with the incorporation of patient satisfaction and access data into the payment scheme. Although this was greeted with protests from practitioners concerned about reliability, early research suggests these fears are exaggerated.[25] However, many patients probably do not fully understand the financial framework that general practice operates within and the extent or effect of payments on the actions of the professionals that care for them. They require more information about the QOF and what scores mean.

POLITICS AND PROFESSIONALISM

The Griffiths reforms of the mid-1980s first introduced private sector management methods into the National Health Service (NHS). In historical terms, from the perspective of policy makers, the QOF represents a high water mark in the onward march of what Harrison has termed 'scientific bureaucratic medicine'. The QOF provides commissioners with, albeit crude, tools for comparing providers as they seek to break the monopolistic stranglehold of traditional general practices in this health sector. There is an irony that Tudor Hart's work on proactive care nearly half-a-century ago may have pre-empted the QOF.[26]

Information technology and electronic records have changed the shape of general practice, not only the way in which medical care is conceived of and delivered but also roles and working routines within practices. The commodification of healthcare via the disaggregation of chronic disease management into itemised, remunerated chunks is a far cry from the professional discretion of yesteryear. Only a generation ago, doctors could hide behind the notion of clinical freedom and the exercise of professional judgement to defend differences in medical decision-making and explain variations in quality of care.[27]

Indicators and guidelines can be a threat to professionalism on three fronts. First, codification into guidelines and the QOF has encouraged external control of clinical practice by 'experts', the National Institute for Health and Clinical Excellence, and indirectly the government that has led to a loss of clinical autonomy. Second, because of the ever increasing knowledge and skills the practitioner has to acquire, the profession has become increasingly fragmented into subspecialties with generalists devolving skills to nurse practitioners and subspecialists such as GPs with special interests.[28] Third, it allows other professionals with narrower areas of knowledge or skills to take over the GP's role such as has occurred with counselling in primary care. This process has also been termed proletarianisation or de-professionalisation.[29]

We are seeing a philosophical shift in which quality of care is being redefined in distinctly limited terms conflated with meeting targets. This is not some postmodern retreat to relativism but an appeal to acknowledge that 'not all that is measurable is of value and that not all that is of value can be measured'. Ironically, many important consequences of the QOF will always elude measurement.

Traditionally, debates between the BMA's 'hoary, battle-hardened trade unionists' and the RCGP's 'ivory-towered academics' over quality improvement were frequently conflictual – especially where remuneration was concerned. In contrast, the negotiations described by Martin Roland conjure up the aura of a gentleman's club. This collaborative endeavour was extremely successful, at least as measured in financial terms for their members. In the longer term, a large price has been and is being exacted as politicians claw back early 'overpayments', most notably through extensions to practice opening hours.

The QOF's continuing development remains an essentially political process. This is nowhere better illustrated than by the fact that all QOF developments for 2009/10 as recommended by the advisory committee were suspended in the wake of the swine flu epidemic as part of bartering over payments to general practices for their part in the swine flu immunisation campaign. What thought in those early days was given to the consequences of underpricing? However, there are attendant dangers for the medical profession. The notion of the 'GP public sector fat cat' has been used to tarnish the image of the profession as a whole, throwing negotiators onto the back foot in times of financial stringency.

A final question for stakeholders ought to concern the environmental sustainability of the QOF. It is helping to drive up process activity such as prescribing rates with detrimental carbon consequences. An environmentally 'steady state' NHS is unlikely given the current drive for change, innovation and efficiency. However, in the health sector as elsewhere, advancement can be achieved without the potentially catastrophic effects of growth on the economy and climate.[30]

WAYS FORWARD

As we look to the future, we should not ignore important lessons from the past. In the confusion over whether the QOF is a quality improvement mechanism or part of a regulatory framework, we should remember that the QOF is part of a wider complex system 'which is perfectly designed to get the results it achieves'.[31] We need ever to be mindful of 'counterfactuals': there are other explanations beyond the QOF for some of the negative consequences we have described. The development of evidence-based medicine,[32] guidelines[33] and organisational changes towards greater skill-mix all predated the QOF, driven by a myriad of policy, regulatory, workforce and other changes. We have grouped concluding comments on future development under four headings:

Limiting the QOF's scale

Despite the QOF being part of the fabric of UK general practice now and in the foreseeable future,[34] inescapable limitations to the evidence base remain, both in terms of the number of areas that can be targeted and the QOFability of indicators. These already impose significant limits on how far and how fast the QOF can be expanded. Lester and Roland have discussed different options for the future development of the QOF (*see* Box 12.1).[35]

Box 12.1 Future options

- Leave indicators unchanged and expect higher achievement each year – restricting the potential benefits of quality measures to a limited number of areas.
- Add new indicators or conditions regularly – could lead to a vast and unmanageable set of measures.
- Build a larger set of evidence-based measures that are all monitored – would measure pay-for-performance against a subset of these.
- Remove measures once a predetermined and agreed level of achievement has been reached – would require robust information about the effect of removing measures.
- Rotate measures regularly, enabling a potential improvement across a range of conditions and areas – would need to be carefully piloted to guard against unintended consequences.

Indeed, there are strong arguments to restrict the proportion of practice pay that is performance-related. Too much money is currently attached to the QOF in the United Kingdom. As several contributors attest, external incentives may lessen motivation – the desire to do a task well for its own sake – if they clash with the professional's perceptions of their role or identity and of quality care.[36] One way forward is to reduce the overall budget for the QOF and ensure that the indicators included are those that are most closely aligned to health professionals' views of their work in primary care.

Increasing public health impact

While the QOF may have contributed in a small way to declining health inequalities, financial incentives need to be firmly realigned to reducing disparities in health provision and outcomes to yield significant progress. In practice, this would mean raising target thresholds on the basis of the remaining percentage performance where, arguably, the greatest health gains are likely to be made and attaching more points (and pounds) to indicators that tackle more significant public health issues.

Thresholds within the QOF need to be set so that there are sufficient incentives for proactive case finding, particularly in deprived areas where disease prevalence rates are higher. Other incentives for staff working in primary care, both financial and non-financial, may improve access for the hard to reach and those with greater healthcare needs.

More research

Unsurprisingly, for all the contributors more research is needed. Nick Steel and Sara Willems laid out the agenda. We need to do more work on the experience and views of patients, users and carers.[37] We should develop better measures for those important aspects of care that are currently not measured or deemed to be 'unmeasurable'. In particular, we need to examine the impact of the QOF on health outcomes and on equity of health outcomes in more detail. Research is also needed in organisational aspects of QOF such as: the weighting of patient-reported experience and outcome measures; how to select new clinical domains and measures for inclusion; effects of 'retiring' indicators from the framework; determining the size of financial rewards and whether reward should be based on workload (as is currently the case) or health outcomes. We have, as yet, little evidence that the QOF represents the most cost-effective approach to improving care among the alternatives that might be available.

Personalizing the QOF

Starfield and Mangin argue that quality initiatives should focus more on adequate recognition of patients' problems, the extent to which patients and practitioners agree on what the patients' problems are, and the degree to which these problems improve over time with medical and other interventions. Personalised advice, informed but not rigidly dictated by evidence, in the context of peoples' lives is indeed the essence of primary care. Treatment must relate to outcomes that are important to the patient. Single disease-based guideline adherence can override respect for patient autonomy and patient welfare. For patients and population groups, co-morbidities are today's norm. Quality initiatives must address the impact of multi-morbidity on life course events, on disability and on polypharmacy.

Can the QOF be developed in a manner that provides informed options for GPs and patients to choose alternatives? Is continuity of care 'QOFable'? A more rational system would allow for flexibility and responsiveness in applying evidence from 'partial statistical lives to complex individual lives'.

Few people in general practice can ignore the magnitude of the QOF's impact on their daily working lives, so perhaps the most telling finding came from Checkland and Harrison. Their interviewees denied major alterations to their practice resulting from the QOF and used the pliable nature of 'holism' to defend rhetorical claims to be providing, unchanged, a patient-centred model of care. It is possible to exaggerate in apocalyptic terms, the QOF's lasting detriment when the outward rituals and routines of daily practice have changed little. General practice has adapted to many different assaults down the decades, but politicians and practitioners alike should be mindful of our testimony in taking the discipline forward.

REFERENCES

1. Sutton M, Elder R, Guthrie B, *et al*. Record rewards: the effects of targeted quality incentives on the recording of risk factors by primary care providers. *Health Econ.* 2010; **19**(1): 1–13.
2. Siriwardena AN. Why do GPs prescribe psychotropic drugs when they would rather provide alternative psychological interventions? *Br J Gen Pract.* 2010; **60**: 241–2.
3. McGinn D, Godman B, Lonsdale J, *et al*. Initiatives to enhance the quality and efficiency of statin and PPI prescribing in the UK: impact and implications. *Expert Rev Pharmacoecon Outcomes Res.* 2010; **10**: 73–85.
4. Alabbadi I, Crealey G, Turner K, *et al*. Statin prescribing in Northern Ireland and England pre and post introduction of the Quality and Outcomes Framework. *Pharm World Sci.* 2010; **32**: 43–51.
5. Belsey J, de Lusignan S, Chan T, *et al*. Abnormal lipids in high-risk patients achieving cholesterol targets: a cross-sectional study of routinely collected UK general practice data. *Curr Med Res Opin.* 2008; **24**: 2551–60.
6. Currie CJ, Peters JR, Tynan A, *et al*. Survival as a function of HbA(1c) in people with type 2 diabetes: a retrospective cohort study. *Lancet.* 2010; **375**: 481–9.
7. Belsey, de Lusignan, Chan, *et al.*, op. cit.
8. Sutton, Elder, Guthrie, *et al.*, op. cit.
9. Walker S, Mason AR, Claxton K, *et al*. Value for money and the Quality and Outcomes Framework in primary care in the UK NHS. *Br J Gen Pract.* 2010; **60**: 213–20.
10. Alsanjari O, van Vlymen J, de Lusignan S. *Pay-for-performance targets distort BP recording: a longitudinal analysis of end digit preference recording in primary care.* Academic Primary Care: Balancing Priorities. London: The Society for Academic Primary Care; 2010.
11. Carey IM, Nightingale CM, Dewilde S, *et al*. Blood pressure recording bias during a period when the Quality and Outcomes Framework was introduced. *J Hum Hypertens.* 2009; **23**(11): 764–70.
12. Edwards A, Langley A. Understanding how general practices addressed the Quality and Outcomes Framework of the 2003 General Medical Services contract in the UK: a qualitative study of the effects on quality and team working of different approaches used. *Qual Prim Care.* 2007; **15**: 265–75.

13. McGregor W, Jabareen H, O'Donnell CA, *et al.* Impact of the 2004 GMS contract on practice nurses: a qualitative study. *Br J Gen Pract.* 2008; **58**: 711–19.
14. Griffiths P, Murrells T, Maben J, *et al.* Nurse staffing and quality of care in UK general practice: cross-sectional study using routinely collected data. *Br J Gen Pract.* 2010; **60**: 36–48.
15. Jamous H, Peloille B. Changes in the French University-Hospital system. In: Jackson JA, editor. *Professions and Professionalisation.* Cambridge: Cambridge University Press; 1970. pp. 111–52.
16. Di Blasi Z, Harkness E, Ernst E, *et al.* Influence of context effects on health outcomes: a systematic review. *Lancet.* 2001; **357**: 757–62.
17. Nazareth I, King M. Decision making by general practitioners in diagnosis and management of lower urinary tract symptoms in women. *BMJ.* 1993; **306**: 1103–6.
18. Naylor CD. Grey zones of clinical practice: some limits to evidence-based medicine. *Lancet.* 1995; **345**: 840–2.
19. Subramanian DN, Hopayian K. An audit of the first year of screening for depression in patients with diabetes and ischaemic heart disease under the Quality and Outcomes Framework. *Qual Prim Care.* 2008; **16**: 341–4.
20. Kendrick T, Dowrick C, McBride A, *et al.* Management of depression in UK general practice in relation to scores on depression severity questionnaires: analysis of medical record data. *BMJ.* 2009; **338**: b750.
21. Byrne PS, Long BEL, Great B; Department of Health and Social Security. *Doctors Talking to Patients: a study of the verbal behaviour of general practitioners consulting in their surgeries.* London: Her Majesty's Stationery Office; 1976.
22. Ritzer G. *The McDonaldization of Society.* 5th ed. Thousand Oaks, CA: Pine Forge Press; 2008.
23. Lester H, Roland M. Future of quality measurement. *BMJ.* 2007; **335**: 1130–1.
24. Baker R, Bankart MJ, Murtagh GM. Do the Quality and Outcomes Framework patient experience indicators reward practices that offer improved access? *Br J Gen Pract.* 2009; **59**: 584–9.
25. Roland M, Elliott M, Lyratzopoulos G, *et al.* Reliability of patient responses in pay for performance schemes: analysis of national General Practitioner Patient Survey data in England. *BMJ.* 2009; **339**: b3851.
26. Hart JT, Thomas C, Gibbons B, *et al.* Twenty five years of case finding and audit in a socially deprived community. *BMJ.* 1991; **302**: 1509–13.
27. Hampton JR. The end of clinical freedom. *Br Med J (Clin Res Ed).* 1983; **287**: 1237–8.
28. Gervas J, Starfield B, Violan C, *et al.* GPs with special interests: unanswered questions. *Br J Gen Pract.* 2007; **57**: 912–17.
29. Siriwardena AN. *Guidelines in Primary Care: an investigation of general practitioners' attitudes and behaviour towards clinical guidelines.* Nottingham: University of Nottingham; 1995.
30. Jackson T. *Prosperity Without Growth: economics for a finite planet.* London: Earthscan; 2009.
31. Nolan TW. Understanding medical systems. *Ann Intern Med.* 1998; **128**: 293–8.
32. Sackett DL, Rosenberg WM. On the need for evidence-based medicine. *J Public Health Med.* 1995; **17**: 330–4.
33. Siriwardena AN. Clinical guidelines in primary care: a survey of general practitioners' attitudes and behaviour. *Br J Gen Pract.* 1995; **45**: 643–7.

34. Lester H, Majeed A. The future of the Quality and Outcomes Framework. *BMJ*. 2008; **337**: a3017.
35. Lester H, Roland H. Measuring quality through performance. Future of quality measurement. *BMJ*. 2007; **335**: 1130–1.
36. Hart, Thomas, Gibbons, *et al.*, op. cit.
37. Adam R. 'Personal Care' and General Practice Medicine in the UK: a qualitative interview study with patients and General Practitioners. *Osteopath Med Prim Care*. 2007; **1**: 13.

Index

Diagrams are given in italics.